Working wi
Self-management
courses
The thoughts of
participants, planners,
and policy-makers

Working with Self-management courses

The thoughts of participants, planners, and policy-makers

Edited by

F. Roy Jones

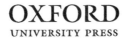

OXFORD
UNIVERSITY PRESS

OXFORD
UNIVERSITY PRESS

Great Clarendon Street, Oxford ox2 6DP

Oxford University Press is a department of the University of Oxford.
It furthers the University's objective of excellence in research, scholarship,
and education by publishing worldwide in

Oxford New York

Auckland Cape Town Dar es Salaam Hong Kong Karachi
Kuala Lumpur Madrid Melbourne Mexico City Nairobi
New Delhi Taipei Toronto

With offices in

Argentina Austria Brazil Chile Czech Republic France Greece
Guatemala Hungary Italy Japan Poland Portugal Singapore
South Korea Switzerland Thailand Turkey Ukraine Vietnam

Oxford is a registered trade mark of Oxford University Press
in the UK and in certain other countries

Published in the United States
by Oxford University Press Inc., New York

British Library Cataloguing in Publication Data

Data available

Library of Congress Cataloguing in Publication Data

Data available

Typeset in Minion by Glyph International, Bangalore, India
Printed in Great Britain
on acid-free paper by the
MPG Books Group, Bodmin and King's Lynn

ISBN 978-0-19-953931-4 (Pbk)

10 9 8 7 6 5 4 3 2 1

In Memory of Bob Sang who died on 5th June 2009.
He was a trusted friend and colleague to many
mentioned in this book.

Bob always maintained:
'Learning to learn together through active listening, real dialogue, and
continuous feedback produces wonderful results: trust, supportive
challenge, and the letting go of self-limiting labels. We are all
fellow citizens – a habit we are learning to regain'.
(From some unpublished musings.)

This book is dedicated to the trainers, tutors, and facilitators whose
energy, integrity, and sensitivity allow people to learn together
to release the talent and creativity through which they can
begin to redefine their futures.

Foreword

Interview with Professor Kate Lorig

Kate Lorig: You sent me a list of things for discussion, but can I start by sharing some news?

The Administration on Ageing, a high-level federal agency in the US, is funding the chronic disease self-management programme in a major way. They originally intended to fund 11 states, but it has risen to most of our states.

Each state does its own thing, but with a coordinating centre in the National Council on Ageing. (The NCOA is somewhat like AGE Concern in the UK.) Nancy Whitelaw, the director of their Center for Healthy Aging, is running this. They not only do work themselves but also subcontract, and we are contracted to support training. This means we develop and provide training at the Trainer of Trainers (T-Trainer) and Master Trainer (MT)[1] levels and run the quality control piece. In 2008, we held 50 trainings in all.

Roy Jones: How did this come about?
KL: It was orchestrated by the NCOA working with government who did 3 or 4 small pilots after the Bush Administration put wording into The Older American Act that they would support evidence-based programmes. Under Secretary of Health, Josephina Carbonell, surveyed federal agencies looking for such programmes and eventually settled on the Chronic Disease Self-Management Programme as one of the programmes they would support. All I had to do was go to the right meetings and smile.

RJ: For newcomers, perhaps we had better go back to some of the basic questions. How many agencies, worldwide are now using the Patient Education Research Center's self-management courses?
KL: The numbers change constantly, but you can check by looking at www.patienteducation.stanford.edu, you can count them under 'Organizations Offering Our Programme'; I think it's about 900 at the moment[2]. How many courses are being delivered under each license varies enormously.

RJ: What self-management courses are now available from Stanford?
KL: There are self-management courses in Arthritis, Chronic Disease, HIV/ AIDS, and Diabetes. A Pain-Management course was developed in Canada,

and by the end of 2009 there will be one for young people with chronic illness developed in Canada and one for Cancer Survivors developed by the Macmillan Cancer Support in England. Courses in development include one for the Severely Mentally Ill being developed at Emory College, Atlanta and there are courses for Obesity being developed in New York City. There are internet courses on Chronic Disease, Arthritis, Diabetes, and Cancer Survivors. We also have an on-line programme for Caregivers funded by the Veterans Administration. We have licensed some of our on-line courses to NCOA and they are now distributing them internationally.

RJ: What is the Patient Education Research Center (PERC) staffing complement now?
KL: Smaller than it was: maybe 8 or 9. We can do so much training because we have been training T-Trainers at the top level. There are 50 or 60 certified to train Master Trainers. When someone wants a training event we arrange it, provide the materials and backstop it, but to actually deliver it, we hire trainers from this expanding resource. It should be noted that some of our courses are available in as many as 15 languages and our Master Trainers and T-trainers also can train in several languages.

RJ: What has been the impact on you and on the work of the unit becoming so international?
KL: It's changed our lives and made things more complicated. Our mission was to develop and evaluate courses and then support fidelity. It was never to support a worldwide movement. We are having to create two units; the larger will focus on the research, the other on the training and technical assistance. I get 3 or 4 emails daily asking for technical assistance, which is time consuming and not what I most want to do. Yes, it has changed the unit.

RJ: How has the balance of agencies delivering courses changed? In the early days hospital staffs seemed to 'get it' but general practice was always a problem.
KL: Well, general practice still doesn't understand it. Really, this is because *self-management* is outside the scope of medical practice. That is partly our fault, because we never attempted to operate in that context, and partly it is the consequence of the funding mechanisms in the US. With few exceptions there is no way of funding this programme within general medicine. Although we haven't had any real opposition from medical practice, it has always been something 'other'. What has happened in the US is that the programme is being distributed through the ageing network.

RJ: At Arthritis Care, Keith Hawley raised hardly any funds from UK health funders but £250,000 from social service providers.

KL: We are very happy to train and help anybody. That simple aim has served us pretty well, because all kinds of people have come our way. Our largest licensee is the Expert Patient Programme-Community Interest Company (EPP–CIC) in England and our smallest, the two disabled women in Seattle who formed a little organization called Winning Turtles. If anybody wants to try something that isn't totally crazy we try to support it. Sometimes it works brilliantly and we have wonderful new collaborators. Sometimes it doesn't work and they go away.

RJ: One of the things that initially attracted me to this work was the congruence between what was being taught and the management approach from Stanford.

KL: Basically, the only thing we do not allow organizations to do is change our programmes without working closely with us. That's because we have always believed in the fidelity of the product.

RJ: But you were fairly tough on conformity in our first year...

KL: And we're still fairly tough. We say to people, 'Of course there have to be changes on the local level, but don't make changes until you've tried it and figured out what you really need to do. Then talk to us'. People start by thinking they are going to have to change so much, but what they actually do is change the foods (for example) and then they talk about it. In both the African American and the Native American communities, there have been additional and different spirituality aspects. With African Americans there is often a prayer before and after a course session and the book contains a spirituality section. With Native Americans the symptom cycle gets changed into a Native American symbol. But these are largely cosmetic changes.

RJ: The basic style of these courses is transcultural.

KL: We worked very hard at making it transcultural or maybe we should say acultural. Let me give you an example. In our Internet programme for diabetes, how do we depict the symptom cycle? We devised something in Stanford and sent it to all the Master Trainers in the world and said, 'This is what we are trying to do. Please make suggestions'. And somebody somewhere came up with the idea of a wagon wheel. Not at all our thought! The beauty of this suggestion is that a wagon wheel can be depicted symbolically in most cultures without having strong emotive ties. It is sort of like a carrot. If you want to use a vegetable known in almost every culture, use a carrot. It is not closely tied to anyone's most important food. We don't always get it right, but asking people seems to work. What makes the programme culturally appropriate is that it is taught by people from a culture to people of their own culture.

RJ: Your doctorate is in Public Health; do you conceive these courses as having a public health significance?

KL: Prevention of infectious disease has always been a key component of public health. Removing the famous pump handle in the East End of London stopped the epidemic of cholera. More recently, public health has had a role in the prevention of chronic illness: The first major campaign was about smoking cessation, Public Health is now is moving to obesity and exercise.

I'm not sure why I still think it is about public health. It's probably a combination of my background and being thrown together with groups of physicians at Stanford Medical School who thought very broadly about chronic disease. Working with Halsted Holman and Jim Fries, I recognized the important insight that most people spend most of their time outside of the health care system, and it occurred to me that we could apply this pubic health model to chronic illness. However, this doesn't fit nicely into either a traditional public health or medical model. The recent initiative by the NCOA is really the first time that the programme has been widely accepted within a public health framework and even then it has been done through *Ageing* not *Health*. More recently, our Centres for Disease Control have put more emphasis on chronic disease self-management.

RJ: Would you agree with me that the UK government was confused as to whether these courses were about condition management or self-management?

KL: I don't know. I was never quite sure why the UK government did what it did. Sir Liam Donaldson, your CMO, felt it was a good idea: it wasn't going to hurt anybody and it was pretty inexpensive. I would love to know why he showed such personal interest in the programme. Its science base meant the scientists wouldn't be too unhappy.

One of the most endearing things that anyone ever did was when I came to London specifically to have dinner with Sir Liam. I got to the hotel and he rang me personally to cancel our meal saying he had something to prepare for the Queen for the following day. I was pretty impressed, but he never let me forget my response, I said this was wonderful because it meant I could go to the ballet instead.

RJ: Can I check a term I've been using since the early days, 'patient education intervention'.

KL: I don't use it any more. When we started 30 years ago, I understood that the words we used were important. *Self-help* was not something we could use, at least in the US, because there was a whole medical self-help movement that had to do with people doing their own medicine. Coming out of the women's liberation movement in Boston it was useful but scared physicians so much that we could not use it. *Patient education* was a term that people knew in those days. However, we chose *self-management* rather than *self-help* because people do in fact manage themselves on a day-to-day basis. The term *self-management* was first used by Tom Creer, a psychologist at the National Jewish Hospital in Denver[3] in the mid 1970s, with asthmatic children. I was not aware of Tom's use of the term when we started, but I think he is the true originator. It's now in general use and I have tried very hard to differentiate it from *patient education* because traditional patient education is focussed on knowledge and behaviours while *self-management* is focussed on outcomes, i.e. reduction of symptoms and more appropriate utilization of health care.

RJ: Can we recap for a moment? How are changes and updates made to existing courses?
KL: Very slowly. We update about every 5 years. If you try to move more quickly, you create havoc round the world. We make use of the 2,500 Master Trainers round the world asking them 'What should we do?' and the suggestions pour in and we add these to the suggestions for improvements that come in weekly. When we are ready, we ask 'What really needs to be changed?' Last time around, it was clear that nobody liked the respiratory pieces in the Chronic Disease Self-Management Course. In both the course manual and the book, people didn't like the nutrition and the communication pieces, so needed changes. Some were small. For example, we were suggesting people drink 8 glasses of fluid a day: we discovered there was absolutely no evidence for that. We'd also been saying people should have protein for breakfast: there's no evidence for that either. We dropped both.

My staff goes through the manual and the book, page by page. If we're unsure, we go back and ask the Master Trainers. A wonderful therapist in Tasmania rewrote the respiration section and just sent it in. I looked at it and shared it with other MTs around the world. We took out some medical elements and then checked with two pulmonologists before we put it in. That's the way it gets done, in an iterative process.

Another weak element was the communications section. So, for a year, we taught our Master Trainers two versions. We told them they could try either version, but to let us know what they thought. The new version was repeatedly reshaped and although I don't think it's right yet, it's much better than it was.

The next edition will have a larger obesity section and also contain references to chronic mental illness.

RJ: Can we explore the place of Albert Bandura's thinking in the work of PERC? If I've got it right the initial arthritis course came out of basic experience, good sense and practice and then Bandura came into the picture and helped systematize the thinking a bit. Am I right?

KL: A lot of it was from common sense, but it also had many elements of social cognitive theory because I was familiar with this. In the original arthritis course, one of the hypotheses in my dissertation was that changes in behaviour would be associated with changes in health status. And that just didn't happen: we could not find a statistical association. We spent a lot of time trying with a lot of high-powered statistical help. So, we did a small study; it may have been one of the earliest I ever had published. We went back to 50 people who had taken the arthritis course. We selected 25 whose (arthritis) pain had got worse and 25 whose pain had improved. We used gerontology students, who were blinded to the fact that we had selected these patients, and said to them, 'Go and find out what on the course they found useful or not useful'. From this piece of qualitative work, it became clear that the people who got worse or to whom nothing happened tended to say, 'Isn't it awful? There's nothing you can do about arthritis'. The other group commonly said that they were more in control. That gave us the clue that we should start looking at control theories.

While I was working on my dissertation I talked to Martin Seligman, the father of 'learned helplessness'. I had some contact with Aron Antonovski who was a visiting scholar at Berkeley when I was there so we looked at congruence theory. And then Susan Folkmann who is one of the mothers of 'stress and coping' theory was also at Berkeley so we looked at that too. However, none of these things seemed very productive. About this time, as we were casting around, Halsted Holman came in saying he'd met someone who might be able to help us. Hal took out a business card and it was Albert Bandura's. It had never occurred to me that Al was on the Stanford campus. I certainly knew his work, but I didn't know he was at Stanford and I had been there 3 or 4 years!

So, we went around and talked to Al Bandura. He is a great man and I was quite impressed. He was intrigued by the problem and curious about the work we were doing. He had a student, Ann O'Leary, who was interested in doing a study on self-efficacy and arthritis. She did her doctoral thesis with us at the same time as Stan Shoore, a Robert Wood–Johnson clinical scholar, developed self-efficacy scales as part of his programme.

Through the years, Al has been incredibly helpful. I think his significance for the work now, is that he established the work as legitimate within psychology. He has been kind enough to put his name on a couple of our publications and he doesn't do this readily. He is a friend and a mentor.

RJ: Can we look at the contribution of different countries? What has the UK contributed to the work generally?
KL: They made it legitimate. Interested people looked at it and said, 'If the NHS wants to do this it cannot be all that bad'. In fact, the second you say that the NHS and (in the US Kaiser Permanente) use this, people take you seriously.

RJ: We have pushed quite hard on the lay-led aspect. How important has that been?
KL: I think in the British context it may have been a mistake. Please don't misunderstand, I do think the course should be lay-led, but allowing it to appear that health professionals were excluded was a step too far. I must be careful because I am making this judgement from afar, and I would not presume to tell anyone what they should do, but health professionals in Britain became alienated because they *perceived* an exclusion whether it was real or not. At Stanford, we are happy to train health professionals. However, if they want to teach, they have to do it in the same way as lay leaders, namely, as volunteers. They get the same training and the same treatment from the unit. About 25% of our leaders are health professionals, most of them with chronic illnesses themselves.

RJ: Do you think the term Expert Patient was helpful?
KL: I think it's an unfortunate term. It reinforced the perception that we won't include health professionals. They felt, rightly, that they had been trained to help people all their lives and now the EPP was telling them they were no good. These two things together were damaging.

RJ: This isn't what we believed.
KL: No, I don't think it is. But when I read the commentary in the BMJ and elsewhere, the writers had no idea what the programme is really about. The commentary had nothing to do with the programme; it had to do with words and perceptions.

RJ: Looking at the British scene it seems that quality control has been pretty variable.

KL: You have a huge and fairly costly system of assessment. I was looking at the cost per course published in an EPP study in 2008 and it is about twice what it costs in the USA. It's a big difference. If you look at (national) economies the outcomes are not very different. However, if you add in assessment costs and still have variability, then those additional cost of outcomes become a really rough judge. It's one of the things we're struggling with in America. Thankfully, the federal study of the system is going to focus hard on fidelity as the courses are used more widely. This is the first time it has been done and may be the main contribution of this big US initiative, because we will learn how to control fidelity.

RJ: Fidelity and quality assurance are important issues.

KL: Yes, but do we *know* that the training has to be done this way or that? We have worked with some assumptions but we don't *know*. We need to know exactly what you need to do to get fidelity.

RJ: What about the Australian contribution?

KL: The Australians did some very different things. They went for a model that was sort of half and half; one health professional and one peer course tutor.

RJ: Didn't they come to self-management by a different route?

KL: Well it's not so different really. It came initially through their Arthritis Foundations.

RJ: Where did the Australian Federal Department of Health and Ageing fit in?

KL: It had been going on long before the DH&A became involved.

RJ: Indeed! It was partly because of Australian newsletters that Arthritis Care became involved here.

KL: They had worked to a very different model keeping their training within the Arthritis Foundation to the exclusion of anyone else. The Arthritis Foundation would only train course tutors and would not give organizations the capacity to run their own programmes. Funding became available from DH&A, but their first Master Training ever in Australia wasn't given until 2007.

RJ: I had never picked that up. So given their particular history what has been their contribution?

KL: By working with Health and Ageing, they have done a pretty decent job of getting the programme out to the agencies. Some, realizing that they could not get Master Training in Australia, came to Stanford. We have trained a lot of Australians.

We should also mention John Belfrage's important work evaluating the CDSMP in four different ethnic communities in Melbourne. Anyone who tries to do this as 4 randomized controlled studies simultaneously has to be out of their mind! And he did it.

RJ: Are there particular contributions from other parts the world?

KL: Yes, I think the people in Shanghai have really shown how to work with a population on a neighbourhood basis. I don't fully understand what Dungbo Fu has done there, but he has done an incredible job very well in a very different society.

Patrick McGowan's work in Canada as far as outreach is concerned is amazing. This programme in British Columbia is quickly spreading east. It has become a programme for four or five provincial governments. Patrick has done this using a largely community-based model and he has been wildly successful, but unfortunately he hasn't published much.

RJ: I wanted to ask about Richard Osborne and Melanie Hawkins work in Melbourne and their idea of a 'response shift'.

KL: If I truly understood 'response shift' this would be easier. Everything is contextual and you 'response shift' all the time. I can 'response shift' you in 10 min. Four years ago the hospital told me I had lymphoma and a couple of days later Hal Holman came over not knowing the diagnosis. He said exactly what is your diagnosis? So, I told him I had large B-Cell lymphoma and he said 'Oh that's great!' and I started crying. Hal suddenly realized that nobody had told me it was a very treatable disease. No cancer is curable, but it is highly treatable. If you're going to have cancer it's a great cancer to have because we have really good medicines for it. My 'response shift' to the disease was instantaneous. So I guess I don't understand the psychometrics well enough.

RJ: I am interested in the research because the majority of published papers show very modest sensible changes and that does not reflect the scale of variations I have encountered.

KL: That's different. You want a 'response shift'. A change in depression is a 'response shift'. The situation, the disease, isn't any different. But one's reaction to the disease is different. I agree with Richard Osborne that we're not capturing all the things that happen to people. One of the reasons we get modest changes is that most interventions identify the specific behaviours and outcomes where you want to achieve changes. However, we are letting people self-tailor their outcomes. Further, if you have a whole slew of people who never have pain, you cannot see big shifts in pain. If you started out on a study where everyone had pain and everybody improved by one point, you'd get a one point shift. If you start out in a study where 50% of the people don't have pain and 50% do, and the 50% with pain move the same one point, you only get half a point change in pain. This happens even more when you add in people with mixed symptoms. It is one of the problems with meta analyses. It took me a long time to appreciate this.

I was reading some beautiful work that Frank Keefe did on arthritis and realized that he doesn't let anyone into his studies that doesn't have a 7 on a 10 point pain scale. Frank gets pretty good changes in pain scores, but he starts with a fairly high score. What he studies is pain: you get huge effect sizes if that is what you are studying. With our studies you are always going to see modest mean changes. There is absolutely nothing wrong with this unless they are brought, with insufficient care, into a meta analysis.

I have just been looking at our diabetes data. We accepted anybody who wanted to join a course. So, if you look at the Spanish diabetes course data and look at the change in haemoglobin HA1C data, the average change is about 0.4; which is not bad. But if you exclude everybody whose haemoglobin HA1C was below 7.0 at outset (normal for diabetes is considered less than 7) and who had never had HA1c above 7, they stayed within a normal range. Then, the HA1C changes are up to 0.7 or 0.8. Someday I am going to publish this because it is something that most researchers don't think about.

RJ: That's an important point that needs to be made very clearly and it's a methodological issue.
KL: True, but then it is poor methodology to segment sample populations so that you get bigger results. That's why we have never done it and sometimes it does not serve us well.

RJ: But if a study is to be comparable with others in the same field, the data has to be comparable.
KL: I totally agree with Richard that we're not capturing everything. I'm not sure his questionnaires are capturing everything either, but he is capturing more.

I think if you really want to capture it you almost have to do it qualitatively. It's almost a Julie Barlow issue. You have to say to people, what is it that happened to you? And then you have to dig.

RJ: Just before we get into Julie's work, I remember you saying to a group of trainers in Scotland in 2000, 'We all know that this is the course that lets us get worse more slowly'.

KL: You are always working against time with this course. The longer your studies go on the more people can say your studies don't hold for 2 years. Well, that's because you make improvements among people that are getting worse. Methodologically, we have done everything with the stats stacked against us. If I really wanted to show ourselves off I would look at 4/5 month studies and I would never look at longitudinal results; and, if I was studying arthritis I would only include people with a pain level above 5 or 6.

RJ: Let's think about Julie Barlow and her unit at Coventry. Much of it is qualitative and is based in Health Psychology.

KL: She does some very nice research that is especially helpful to academia and theory.

RJ: So, the strength of the work Julie has done lies in the strength of the work itself.

KL: Yes and she has informed us about how to strengthen the courses and who benefits from these interventions.

RJ: Finally, are there contributions from religion? From Judaism, Christianity or Islam?

KL: I haven't given this enough thought to be able to give you a cogent answer. Probably yes, but not in the sense that we're trying to convert anybody. Ben Franklin said that God helps those that help themselves. Hillel said that 'If I am not for myself, who will be? If I am only for myself, what am I? And if not now, when?' (Pirkei Avot 1:14) There is certainly a lot of tradition there.

Endnotes

1 T-Trainers are the senior, highly trained and experienced trainers who are licensed to train Master Trainers and can operate within and between agencies.

2 This chart shows the license holders worldwide. The numbers delivering or receiving training vary widely. However the chart does give an indication of the international penetration at 21 May 09. The website also shows the names by which courses are known locally. 'Healthier Living' is a popular alternative to CDSMC in the 40 Kaiser Permanente licensees.

	English Chronic Disease course	Spanish Chronic Disease course	HIV/AIDS course	Arthritis course	Spanish Arthritis course
USA	546	84	32	27	14
Argentina		1			1
Australia	86			8	
Austria	1				
Barbados				1	
Canada	86		1	1	
China & Hong Kong	10			2	
Chile		1			
Columbia		1			
Denmark	1				
Holland	2				
Ireland	2				
Italy	2				
Japan	2		1		
Korea	1				
Lithuania				1	
Mexico		7			1
New Zealand	3			1	
Northern Ireland	4				
Norway	6				
Peru		1			
Singapore	2				
South Africa	1				
South Korea	1				
Spain	1	2			1
St Lucia	1			1	
Sweden	2				
Switzerland	1				
Taiwan	1				
UK	15		4	2	

3   Kate R. Lorig, Halsted R. Holman, Stanford University School of Medicine, *Annals of Behavioral Medicine* 2003, vol 26, No. 1, pp. 1–7. Self-Management Education: History, Definition, Outcomes, and Mechanisms.

Contents

Contributors

Phil Baker
Operations Director,
Arthritis Care
London

Julie Barlow, Ph.D., B.A.
Chartered Health Psychologist,
Professor of Health Psychology,
Coventry University

Elizabeth Bayliss
Executive Director, Social Action for
Health, Tower Hamlets

**David Colin-Thomé, OBE, MB, BS,
FRCGP, FFPH, FRCP**
National Clinical Director for
Primary Care (England),
Department of Health

Jane Cooper, M.Sc., B.Sc.
Talking Health Network
Ramsgate

Christine E. A. Cupid
Course Tutor, Social Action for
Health, Tower Hamlets

Angela Donaldson, M.A.
Director, Arthritis Care in Scotland
Glasgow

**Ayesha Dost, Ph.D., M.S., M.BA.,
M.A., B.A. (Hons)**
Director, Self Care Support Global;
formerly: Policy Adviser,
Department of Health

**Natalie Grazin, M.A. (Oxon),
M.A., M.PA.**
Assistant Director,
The Health Foundation
London

Kathy Hawley, M.A., Ph.D.
Independent Consultant; Research
and Development
Oxford

Keith Hawley, M.A. (Oxon)
Business Development and
Partnership Consultant
Oxford

Patrick Hill, C. Psychol
Professional Lead Clinical Health
Psychology, NHS Birmingham East
and North

Barbara Hogg
Self-Management Tutor,
Northamptonshire,
Arthritis Care

F. Roy Jones, M.Min., DMS
Independent Consultant, Manchester
Formerly Director of Services
Arthritis Care

Anne Kennedy, Ph.D., B.Sc., SRN
Senior Research Fellow,
The National Primary Care Research
and Development Centre,
University of Manchester

Simon Knighton
Chief Executive, The Expert Patients
Programme Community Interest
Company

Kate Lorig, Dr. PH, RN
Professor, Director of the Patient
Education Research Center,
Stanford University School of
Medicine, Palo Alto, California

Carol McNaughton
Course Tutor, Glasgow,
Arthritis Care, Scotland

Ian McNeil, M.A., Chartered MCIPD
Independent Consultant
Inverness

Jennifer Newbould, Ph.D., B.Sc.
Analyst RAND Europe, formerly
Research Fellow, The School of
Pharmacy, London University

Mike Osborn
Consultant Macmillan Clinical
Psychologist, Royal United Hospital,
Bath NHS Trust

Jim Phillips, B.A.
Director of Product Development &
Quality, Expert Patient Programme
Community Interest Company,
Bath

Anne Rogers, Ph.D, M.Sc., B.A., SRN
Professor of the Sociology of
Health Care, Head of Primary Care
Research Group,
University of Manchester

Bob Sang, B.A. (Hons)
Professor of Patient and Public
Engagement on Health, London
South Bank University (deceased)

David G. Taylor, Ph.D., B.Sc., FFPH
Professor of Pharmaceutical and
Public Health Policy,
The School of Pharmacy,
London University

Jean Thompson, MBE, B.A.
DipCounselling, DipVG, Talking
Health Network,
Ramsgate

Andy Turner, B.Sc., Ph.D.
Senior Research Fellow, Applied
Research Centre in Health &
Lifestyle Interventions
Coventry University

Course Tutor
The Christie, Manchester
(Personal details withheld)
Queries via Gail Neillings,
EPP Co-ordinator
The Christie, Manchester

**Louise Wallace, Ph.D., M.BA., B.A.
(Soc Sci) Psychology**
Professor of Psychology and Health,
Coventry University

Chapter 1

UK origins and arguments

F. Roy Jones

In one way or another, every contributor to this book has had an involvement with the self-management courses developed at Stanford University. I believe that by bringing these together they illuminate each other and enable readers to develop a comprehending grasp of what has been learned to date. We started with a foreword by Kate Lorig because it all began in 1978 when she commenced her studies for a doctorate in public health. Today, Kate is a full professor in Stanford Medical School and is still a little surprised that this is where a nursing student with an interest in obstetrics and gynaecology has ended up. All the rest of us have been involved in some way since these courses arrived in the UK in 1993. The book is neither a history nor an uncritical advocacy. It is rather a multi-faceted and layered look that allows readers to 'get it' when the subject is being discussed and make their own evaluation of the main ideas.

In her foreword, Kate Lorig introduced herself and Stanford's Patient Education Research Center (PERC) where she is the director. In a 2001 paper[1], she outlined five core self-management skills: 'problem solving, decision making, resource utilization, forming a patient/health care provider partnership, and taking action'. In this book, the term self-management usually contains these five dimensions. It is important to note that these are not primarily about chronic diseases, but the skills that equip people to live with chronic diseases and perceive a substantial degree of control. At core, these courses are more about managing self than the disease.

The first course developed at PERC, and indeed the first delivered in the UK was the Arthritis Self-Management Course (ASMC) styled by Arthritis Care *Challenging Arthritis*. This 'patient education intervention' (as then known) was designed as an exercise in peer learning. Logically, therefore, both participants and volunteer course tutors should share some basic features. In this case, experience of arthritis. Since rheumatological conditions do not discriminate and are very common, there are plenty of skilled people to draw upon and, in California and the UK, many of the earliest volunteer course tutors had professional health or educational backgrounds. They always conducted the course in pairs. Each 'course' has six sessions, one per week, each of two hours with a half hour break. In those early days, quite an effort was made to avoid using venues where participants go for treatment. Pubs, community centres, private houses, and shopping centres were all tried in order to convey the core idea that this course is about what participants can do themselves.

Not everyone in the US or the UK welcomed these innovative courses. But in both places, it was the charity sector that seized their potential. Some doctors and other health professionals, who play major roles in health related charities, were suspicious of a course that ran without their rightful involvement, professional oversight, guarantee of legitimacy, and patient safety. That 'patients' could go on to train to become course tutors and deliver these courses seemed suspect. However, the burst of activism within Arthritis Care that followed the introduction of these courses added to the pressure for organizational change and argued for greater participation by people with arthritis in governance. After initial reluctance, the Medical Advisory Committee at Arthritis Care, chaired by Dr. David Doyle, encouraged their development and helped to appoint a research advisory group that worked with Julie Barlow (now professor) on Coventry University's initial evaluation when project funding was secured.

At the beginning of her studies, Kate Lorig had spent a month exploring the experiences of people with arthritis living in the community: there, she discovered a largely untapped resource of problem-solving skill. This, together with the realization that patients need not know a great deal of rheumatology to be able to cope effectively, informed her work devising the prototype self-management course. In 1996/1997, just as Challenging Arthritis was settling down in the UK (and especially well in Scotland), PERC took the next logical step and trialled a new course stripped of disease specific content. The research was published in 1998. This was the Chronic Disease Self-Management Course (CDSMC) that became the foundation for work in the UK, Australia, around the globe, and, somewhat belatedly, the USA.

Richard Osborne took over from Jean Gaffin as Arthritis Care's CEO (1995–2001) and enthusiastically supported her initiatives with Challenging Arthritis and with Long-term Conditions Alliance[2] (LMCA). He and Judy Wilson, the new CEO of LMCA, encouraged debate among its member organizations resulting in several becoming involved in the long-term illness project (affectionately known as Lill) headed by Jane Cooper. Many organizations discovered this within their memberships too, there were unacknowledged resources of problem-solving skill. For the first time, the CDSMC embraced people experiencing psychiatric symptoms (viz. the Manic Depression Fellowship,

The Bipolar Organization). They had recently discovered, when many members brought posters showing how they avoided slipping into mania, that they too had a plethora of problem-solving techniques available. The MDF subsequently developed, and continues to deliver, its own programme.

Quality grant making is a little acknowledged art, but without the expertise of the Smith Charity, the slow start up and exponential growth of Arthritis Care's programme would have been impossible. Smith required a letter of support from the DH and a research component. In time, the Scottish National Lottery Charities Board was similarly helpful. Gradually, Richard Osborne's insight that 'the charities that survive will be those with services that someone wishes to purchase' prevailed. Section 64 funding provided a thrust to secure service delivery agreements. And pharma played a significant role. Searle (now absorbed into Pfizer) initially saw support for Challenging Arthritis as adding value to the Arthrotec brand they were promoting. However, they came to see that there was an additional benefit. Self-managing people use medications deliberately, as a part of their toolkit for managing their condition, not as magic bullets that remove the problem. A number of GP practices began to relate via an initiative promoted by Searle representatives.

PERC's courses are similar anywhere in the world ensured by licensing agreements. Course and programme titles vary, but a fundamental similarity is preserved and people from different cultures readily exchange experience and use compatible, activity focused vocabularies. A London trainer said, 'We don't do sympathy'. Trainers everywhere would know what she meant.

Overview

In the next chapter, Jenny Newbould describes the wider social and health care contexts in which the self-management phenomenon emerged. She confronts the policy issues and draws attention to the new tasks in a rapidly changing context.

Chapter 3 provides three accounts from course participants illustrating the profound influence these courses have on some people. While accounts of rigorous qualitative and quantitative studies wait for Chapter 12, these activist accounts are a true starting point. Arthritis Care was unprepared for the release of energy that sprang from people who attended the initial courses in 1993/1994, but it set out to deliver an integrated programme to empower and support people with arthritis. This was no ambitious paradigm for new service delivery, rather it had equality values and purposes woven into the way in which the course tutors are recruited, trained, and delivered courses. Their very part-time managers (Self-Management Trainers) provided leadership and embraced role modelling. This was characteristic of the hierarchical structure developed in the programme. SMT and tutor training events were delivered by Jean Thompson (now MBE) after her Master Training course at Stanford.

In Chapter 4, the insights of three very different tutor trainers are provided. Barbara Hogg's contribution is the most personal; as one of the original intake of tutors still practising, she takes the long view, describing her journey with the unusual addition of a contribution from Adult Education. Today, Kathy Hawley and Andy Turner are academic developer/researchers, but were in previous lives, respectively, a social worker and a professional footballer. Kathy's initial involvement was writing internal management reports for Arthritis Care. More recently, she wrote a course with young people. The subsequent EPP course Live Positively won EPP a Guardian award for innovation. Andy was part of Julie Barlow's research team in Challenging Arthritis' early days. Still working with the CDSMC and the Co-Creating Health project, he has gone on to develop the HOPE course working up the ideas in the context of mental health.

In Chapter 5, Jean makes a powerful case that is at odds with many current initiatives. She rues the loss of the special cadre of people with long-term conditions who found energy together both in developing voluntary sector and NHS services. Her programme emphasis was on the commonality of the experience of developing a long-term condition. Everyone comes to such a diagnosis unprepared and is at that moment 'lay'. Jean explores the value of this approach and rails against the professionalization of some new initiatives.

The variety and modes of organization and service delivery are thoroughly explored in Chapter 6. Jim Phillips, at the Expert Patients Programme-Community Interest Company (EPP–CIC) surveys what is being achieved in England. This is in striking contrast with Angela Donaldson's[3] very different Scottish perspective. Here, scale issues come into bolder relief: Is smaller government better able to work with these insights? The potential of course delivery by internet is discussed by Ian McNeil who conducted the UK study for Stanford. Up to this point, we have been largely concerned with the move towards service delivery by state agencies. Phillip Baker[4] takes a different view, examining the contribution of voluntary and community agencies. His points are substantially supported by Elizabeth Bayliss from her experience with a mixed and predominately Bengali community in Tower Hamlets. Jane Cooper completes the chapter by refocusing the discussion on quality. As an issue, this has been just below the surface in many of the contributions and may be elucidated by the new work in America. It remains an issue as research and evaluation take centre stage.

There has been active debate about what happens to course participants ever since the initial publication of Kate's findings. What outcomes reflect personal experience and what collective? What are culturally determined and what are universal? What depends on the quality of the presentation and the quality of the course design? One of the NHS Clinical Governance Team, Dr. Patrick Hill working with Mike Osbourn, explores this and the experiences of a number of individuals in Chapter 7. The conventional way of assessing a person considers their self-esteem to be central. Interestingly, this approach is dissonant with the self-efficacy approach pioneered by Albert Bandura that looks primarily at the individual's self-efficacy in a specified area. This difference may have significance for the discussion because of its impact on the behaviour of health professionals.

The term Expert Patients was coined by Sir Liam Donaldson who gave it a wide meaning. In addition to the meanings already defined by Kate Lorig (above), it also carries the conviction that some GPs still tend to patronize their patients and fail to capitalize on their abilities in the management of their long-term conditions. The early course protocols advised participants to tell their GPs that they were doing an education course and sought their support. Some GPs were content, but others were suspicious about another new thing from California, that hotbed of wild ideas. Those that immediately saw the point and enjoyed the benefits of working with it supported the attitude and policy developed by the Department of Health. In Chapter 8, David Colin-Thome provides his and the DH's view of the way in which self-management courses fit into the wider policy framework of 'supported self care' initiatives.

A feature of Arthritis Care's work by the new millennium was the high proportion of funding for self-management courses secured by service agreements with local authority Social Service departments. This aspect had dropped below the horizon, but is picked up by Keith Hawley in Chapter 9. He found that directors of social services understood the objectives and methodologies more readily than PCT commissioners and executives. The role of social services as advisors to clients on the management of their health care is an area of debate and controversy, but it seems possible that the cultural and educational thought forms implicit in self-management are more readily embraced in social than in medical care (still dominated by acute care models of intervention). There may be an issue for research methodology here. The double-blinded cross over randomized control study is the gold standard for time limited reversible interventions. But educational interventions are not reversible, and no one doubts that their consequences can be life changing.

The interview with Ayesha Dost[5] reported in Chapter 10 is a revelation. Ayesha was charged with managing the first stage of the Expert Patients Report recommendations (2001) by providing a taster experience for every PCT in England (then 303 bodies). Numerically, this required the appointing sufficient staff to provide cover to all the PCTs in each Strategic Health Authority area. Perhaps for the first time ever the NHS included personal experience of chronic disease in a job description. Highly qualified people applied for these posts. Their task was to animate each PCT into recruiting and training volunteers who would provide at least nine courses in each PCT. This would allow PCTs to learn from the novel experience of working in this way. A small amount of money was allocated to each PCT to finance the experiment. Ayesha uses a learning points approach to describe her learning and unique perspective and analysis to the emergence of the EPP.

In Chapter 11, the struggle to implement the public and patient engagement policies issues are addressed by Professor Bob Sang and Alf Collins. The potential of self-management 'graduates' is apparent to anyone who has spent time with them; not least because a good proportion are keen to contribute their time and skills to the care of others. However, few PCTs are used to organising and deploying volunteers except in highly prescribed roles and these people are independent minded. There should be a ready link between this articulate resource and the policies developed, but it is not easy to create in state bodies.

In Chapter 12, Natalie Grazin[6] introduces the Co-Creating Health project and points to the innovations they have introduced, asserting the significance of working with the NHS because of its dominant influence in the UK understanding of health and health care.

Chapter 13 is the most academic and covers a lot of ground. It is self-evident that when academics conduct studies, they develop a profound familiarity with their subjects. However, they are only rarely asked what they learned beyond the formal structures of their researches. Professors Anne Rogers,[1] Julie Barlow, and Louise Wallace have been asked to do just this in addition to summarizing the findings of their studies. The studies begun by Julie Barlow soon after she obtained her doctorate became one of the building blocks for the work of Applied Research Centre in Health and Lifestyle Interventions Department's work in Coventry. There are many studies now in the catalogue. The largest single study was conducted by Anne Rogers' team and collaborators from York and Bristol, at the Primary Care Research and Development Unit at Manchester University. This work was well disseminated through a series of seminars chaired by Chris Ham. The other building block at Coventry was laid by Louise Wallace bringing the experience of running a PCT. Her team has worked on The Health Foundation's programme Co-Creating Health.

There are layers of discussion behind many apparently obvious initiatives, and behind the scenes there had been conversations involving Stephen Thornton the CEO of The Health Foundation that led to exploratory papers, for example from Ann Coulter at the Picker Institute, resulting in the formulation of the Co-Creating Health project. These recognized that the roll out of the EPP had lacked integration with health professionals and policy directors.

By Chapter 14, so much has been said about the EPP and so many have done work for, or been employed by the EPP–CIC that the contribution from Simon Knighton seems long overdue. The scale of the government inspired initiative programme is reviewed and its prospectus laid out.

Where do these programmes belong? Are they part of a necessary transformation within a sometimes unresponsive health service? David Taylor was the only senior academic present when Sir Liam Donaldson launched the Expert Patients Report in 2001. Chapter 15's title 'Hard Talk is borrowed from 'BBC News 24 Hours' series. Here David looks critically at what has been said and takes a view of the contributions. In particular, he frames these in the context of the policy debates and processes currently underway, poses some challenging questions and sharpens the issues.

Finally in Chapter 16, I attempt to draw out a few major insights from my perspective. I have lived with these concerns for over 15 years and there are tensions and issues that I feel still need to be addressed, but in a new way.

Acknowledgements

There is so much more to be said than it has been possible to encompass in these pages. To all the people who have contributed to my enjoyment and delight in this field, my heartfelt thanks. I wish more of you could be named here but without adding contexts that would have added little. When working for Arthritis Care the threesome of Jean Thompson, Keith Hawley driving these ideas forward was so stimulating. But more recently there have been many other conversations and they lie behind the chapters that follow. The conversation in Tower Hamlets that persuaded Christine Cupid to put pen to paper was great fun. The discovery that Arthritis Care staff colleagues in Scotland were meeting in their offices on the day I met with their director, Angela Donaldson, was exciting. Their experience is so different from the English. The hours interviewing Kate Lorig, Ayesha Dost, Natalie Grazin and Bob Sang were all inspiring. To these, I have to add special mention of the colleagueship and challenge of David Taylor and Jenny Newbould in London, and Julie Barlow and Louise Wallace with their staff teams at Coventry. My family, perforce perhaps, has been very patient with me, and the constant support of my partner Rosemary Beeson, has been invaluable, proof reading all the text even when I could no longer distinguish the wood from the trees.

Finally but not least, OUP's editor Nic Ulyatt and her assistant, Jenny Wright, had, I think, the measure of my inexperience long before I recognised its limitations. They have been patient and forward thinking throughout.

Endnotes

1 *Self-management Education, context, definition and outcomes, and mechanisms.* Kate Lorig Dr. PH, RN, and Halsted Holman, MD, Stanford University School of Medicine. (Parts of this paper were presented at the first Chronic Disease Self-Management Conference, Sydney Australia August, 2000.)

2 Now re-badged as National Voice.

3 Policy and Campaign's Manager at Arthritis Care, Scotland.

4 Operations Manager at Arthritis Care, England.

5 Principal Analyst and Policy Adviser at the Department of Health.

6 Assistant Director for Supporting Patients at The Health Foundation.

Chapter 2

The ideas and health context from which self-management emerged

Jennifer Newbould

In the last hundred years, the health issues of the UK population have been transformed dramatically. Changes in demographic and epidemiological transition (1) have led to alterations in health patterns in the UK and other developed countries. Conditions which used to cause death, such as smallpox, have largely been eliminated and rates of infant mortality have greatly reduced. With increased life expectancy, and therefore a larger elderly population, there has been an expansion in the number of people living with long-term conditions.

These changes in the nature of illnesses suffered by the population have meant health care practices have had to be adapted. Care has shifted from being primarily in hospitals towards the provision of care within the community. This is particularly evident in the case of mental health where care within asylums has been replaced by care in community settings.

Much has been written regarding sociological approaches to the study of illness. One of the earliest approaches, in the 1950s, was Talcott Parsons' 'sick role' (2) that outlined a temporary state in which an ill person was exempt from normal social roles and obligations, such as work, and was able to adopt a 'sick role'. Gallagher's (3) critique of Parsons stated that it is more suited to acute rather than chronic illness, as individuals are not able to be exempt from social roles indefinitely.

Strauss' (4) work emphasized that managing a chronic illness was not just a medical issue, but a social one too. He noted the effects of a condition on an individual's family or partner and the management involved in living with a chronic condition, such as controlling symptoms and overseeing treatment regimens. Other authors have also drawn attention to the considerable role of family members in managing chronic illness (5, 6, 7).

Strauss' (4) view of the effort involved in managing a chronic condition was also noted by Corbin and Strauss (8, 9). They identified three lines of work undertaken by those with chronic illnesses:

+ Illness work (e.g. managing the condition and symptoms)

+ Everyday life work (housework, looking after children)

+ Biographical work (reconstruction of the individual's biography)

Self-management programmes may be seen to reflect this shift away from an individual being exempt from normal roles due to their condition towards managing their condition in the context of their life. The work of Bury (10–12) in this area has emphasized the impact of chronic illness on the biography of the individual. Those diagnosed with a chronic illness go through stages of illness experience; onset, the impact of treatment and the development of adaptive resources. People learn to cope with their condition and develop strategies to limit the effects of the illness. They may also develop individual coping styles to adapt to their condition(s).

The effect of chronic illness on an individual's body has also been the focus of study with links drawn between the body and identity in illness. Charmaz (13) describes how those with a chronic condition experience a 'loss of self', a state that later work suggests individuals may be able to overcome (14). Kelly and Field (15) note that while the body is usually taken for granted when a person is well, if they have a chronic condition their body 'malfunctions' and affects the individual's sense of self and relationship with society.

The writings of medical sociologists have however been contentious to some with disabilities (16). Since the 1960s, there have been differences of opinion between these two groups who take different viewpoints on the issue of disability. Disability and living with a long-term condition are categories that frequently overlap.

Early exponents of the disability movement conveyed an assertive approach to disability. Their view was of disability as a form of social oppression (17); in essence, it is the society that disables people rather than their medical condition. The formation of the Union of the Physically Impaired Against Segregation (UPIS) in 1972 by Vic Finkelstein and Paul Hunt promoted the notion of 'the social model of disability' (18):

> *In our view, it is society which disables impaired people. Disability is something imposed on top of our impairments by the way we are unnecessarily isolated and excluded from full participation in society.*

(UKPIAS, 1975)

The views reported in Hunt's (19) book on stigma were reflected in a wider focus on the disadvantages and discrimination suffered by those with disabilities and the view that disabled people were excluded and oppressed by society. Disability became a political cause, taken up in a fashion similar to campaigns against sexism or racism.

Thomas (20) has argued that the viewpoints of medical sociologists and disability campaigners may not be as disparate as was once believed, with common ground shared underneath these different approaches. It could be argued that disability discrimination acts have sought to reduce societal prejudice. Most recently (the act of 1995 and the subsequent act of 2005) in relation to disability secured rights of employment, education, and access to facilities and transport.

Against the backdrop of these debates, Kate Lorig at Stanford University in the US developed the Arthritis Self-Management Programme (ASMP) a self-management programme for people with arthritis whose tutors were volunteers. Lorig's early published work noted that there was little difference in outcome measures between self-management courses delivered by health professionals compared to those administered by non-professionals (21).

It should be noted that the concept of self-management was not a new phenomenon; people with chronic conditions routinely manage their own conditions, monitor symptoms, manage medication, and adapt lifestyles. Nor was the development of a group environment for those with chronic conditions a novel approach, charity organizations have for many years run support groups for those with chronic conditions. The ASMP approach was distinct from most other self-management interventions which seek to impart technical knowledge or skills to manage a specific condition in the use of lay, rather than professional, tutors.

From the ASMP, Lorig became aware that many participants had not only a diagnosis of arthritis but also other chronic conditions too. This observation led to the development, during the 1990s, of a generic chronic disease self-management programme (CDSMP) suitable for those with any chronic condition and those with co-morbidities (22). Today, the CDSMP is used in over 20 countries around the world, most notably the US and Australia, and has been translated into numerous languages. Although the basic course is used, culturally sensitive modifications are made. For example, for Chinese cultures it was deemed inappropriate to discuss death and this section of the course was deleted (23).

The CDSMP has also been developed in formats other than face-to-face group meetings, for example, mail delivered courses in arthritis (24), an internet-based back pain programme (25) and internet-based course for those with HIV (26). The course has also been adapted for carers, parents/guardians, young people, and those with communication difficulties.

Despite the growth in the generic course, attention has been drawn in more recent years to the need to develop condition-specific courses (27). These include those for back care and diabetes, and courses targeted to specialized groups such as those with chronic conditions who wish to return to work, people living with alcohol and drug dependency and those with chronic conditions in prison (28).

In the UK, the development of EPP emerged from a number of Government policies. In 1999, the Chief Medical Officer, Sir Liam Donaldson, set up a task force to design a new EPP (29):

> to address the needs of the very many people in this country with a chronic disease or disability, who amount to one in three of the total population.

> (Department of Health, 1999)

It was later estimated that ten million people in England were living with a chronic condition (30).

The EPP formally began in 2001. The term 'Expert Patient' may have subsequently discouraged people from the organization, fearing that patients must, as a requirement, have large amounts of knowledge about their condition. In selecting the term, Donaldson advocated the name to reflect the patient as an 'expert and partner in their care' (30).

The NHS Improvement Plan (31) included a chapter entitled 'supporting people with long-term conditions to live healthy lives'. This reported how the use of trained non-medical leaders could equip those with chronic conditions with the skills to manage their own conditions. Although not implicit in the Government documents, it should be noted that the development of lay-led self-management policies in the UK have emerged at a time of concern over NHS spending and health care costs. Due to delivery by lay leaders, the EPP delivers a relatively cost effective (32) intervention for those with chronic conditions.

Further Government publications have emphasized the importance of the management of chronic conditions (33, 34). In 2006, the White Paper on community services outlined the Government's commitment to treble its investment in the EPP to support the transfer of the EPP to a Community Interest Company (CIC). In the pilot phase, the EPP was nationally funded. From 2007, it has been a CIC. It can be commissioned directly by PCTs and GPs and stands outside the NHS.

Looking to the future of the EPP, Kennedy et al. (2004) (26) warn of the need to manage the risk of EPP becoming marginalized rather than mainstreamed. The most recent reports have recommended the EPP to be more flexible to meet the needs of different groups (35). Alongside this is the evident need to continue recruiting participants and volunteers to the courses. In the UK pilot study, 17% of Primary Care Trusts (PCTs) that participated had not completed any course in the target period (26). A failure, in the main, to engage support from health professionals, particularly GPs, means many people with chronic conditions may be unaware of the existence of the EPP.

It is clear from talking to people who have participated in EPP courses that the experience has the potential to change their emotional well-being and ability to manage their condition. However, there is still a lack of evidence which demonstrates this to be so (36), nor a comprehensive understanding of how sustained such improvements are. Recruiting fewer participants who are male (37) or from ethnic minorities (38) may not be indicative of a failure to engage these groups. Rather that, while the lay-led approach to the management of chronic conditions is preferred by some, it may not be suited to all. Individuals who face the challenges of a chronic condition may choose to cope in a different way. These issues are discussed in the following chapters of this book. It is my view that those who benefit from the EPP should be able to continue to do so. Provision should be part of a range of resources, such as those from the voluntary sector, which reflect the different requirements of varied members of the community.

References

1. Taylor D., Bury M. (2007) Chronic illness, expert patients and care transition. *Sociology of Health & Illness.* **29**(1): 27–45.
2. Parsons T. (1951) *The Social System.* Glencoe: Free Press.
3. Gallagher E. (1976) Lines of reconstruction and extension in Parsonian sociology of illness. *Social Science and Medicine.* **10**: 207–18.
4. Strauss A. (1973) America: In sickness and in health. *Society.* **19**: 33–9.
5. Anderson R. (1988) The quality of life of stroke patients and their carers. In: Anderson R and Bury M (editors) *Living with Chronic Illness: the Experiences of Patients and Their Families.* London: Unwin Hyman.
6. Canam C. (1993) Common adaptive tasks facing parents of children with chronic conditions. *Journal of Advanced Nursing.* **18**: 46–53.
7. Jobling R. (1988) The experience of psoriasis under treatment. In: Anderson R and Bury M (editors) *Living with Chronic Illness: the Experiences of Patients and their families.* London: Unwin Hyman.
8. Corbin J., Strauss AL. (1985) Managing chronic illness at home: three lines of work. *Qualitative Sociology.* **8**: 224–47.
9. Corbin J., Strauss A. (1988) *Unending Work and Care: Managing Chronic Illness at Home.* San Francisco: Josey Bass.
10. Bury M. (1982) Chronic illness as biographical disruption. *Sociology of Health and Illness.* **4**(2): 167–82.

11. Bury M. (1988) Meanings at risk: the experience of arthritis. In: Anderson R., Bury M. (editors) *Living with Chronic Illness: the Experiences of Patients and Their Families*. London: Unwin Hyman.

12. Bury M. (1991) The sociology of chronic illness: a review of research and prospects. *Sociology of Health and Illness*. 13(4): 451–68.

13. Charmaz K. (1983) Loss of self: a fundamental form of suffering in the chronically ill. *Sociology of Health and Illness*. 5(2): 168–95.

14. Charmaz K. (2000) Experiencing chronic illness. In: Albrecht GL, Fitzpatrick R, Scrimshaw SC (editors) *The Handbook of Social Studies in Health and Medicine*. London: Sage.

15. Kelly M., Field D. (1996) Medical sociology, chronic illness and the body. *Sociology of Health and Illness*. 18: 241–57.

16. Barnes C., Mercer G. (editors) (1996) *Exploring the Divide: Illness and Disability*. Leeds: The Disability Press.

17. Abberley P. (1987) The concept of oppression and the development of a social theory of disability. *Disability and Society*. 2(1): 5–19.

18. UKPIAS (1975) *Union of the Physically Impaired Against Segregation Comments on the discussion held between the Union and the Disability Alliance on 22nd November, 1975*. Available from http://www.leeds.ac.uk/disability-studies/archiveuk/finkelstein/UPIAS%20Principles%202.pdf [accessed 7th July 2009].

19. Hunt P. (1966) *Stigma: The Experience of Disability*. London: Geoffrey Chapman.

20. Thomas C. (2004) How is disability understood? An examination of sociological approaches. *Disability and Society*. 19(6): 569–83.

21. Lorig K., Feigenbaum P., Regan C., et al. (1986) A comparison of lay-taught and professional-taught arthritis self management courses. *Journal of Rheumatology*. 13 (4): 763–7.

22. Sobel DR., Lorig KR., Hobbs, M. (2002) Chronic disease self-management programme: from development to dissemination. *The Permanente Journal*. 6(2): 15–22.

23. Fu D., Fu F., McGowan P., et al. (2003) Implementation and qualitative evaluation of chronic disease self management programmeme in Shanghai, China: a randomized controlled trial. *Bulletin of the World Health Organization*. 81(3): 174–82.

24. Lorig KR., Ritter PL., Laurent DD., Fries JF. (2004) Long-term randomized controlled trial of tailored-print and small-group arthritis self-management interventions. *Medical Care*. 42(4): 346–54.

25. Lorig K., Battersby M. (2003) The Integration of chronic condition self-management into health systems - a world view. Paper presented at *Guiding Us Forward the National Chronic Condition Self-Management Conference*, 12–14 November 2003, Melborne, Australia.

26. Stanford University (2005) Available at http://patienteducation.stanford.edu/programmes/psmp.html [accessed on 8 May 2005].

27. Kennedy, A., Gately, C., Rogers, A., EPP evaluation team (2004) National evaluation of expert patients programmeme; Assessing the process of embedding EPP in the NHS, Preliminary survey of PCT pilot sites. National Primary care research and development centre; Manchester.

28. Expert Patients Programme (EPP) (2008) Progress Report. Available from <http://www.expertpatients.co.uk/public/cms/uploads/ProgressReport08.pdf? [Accessed 16th July 2009).

29. Department of Health (1999) *Saving Lives: Our Healthier Nation*. London: Stationary Office.

30. Donaldson L. (2003) Expert patients usher in a new era of opportunity for the NHS. *British Medical Journal.* **326**: 1279–80.

31. Department of Health (2004) *The NHS Improvement Plan: Putting People at the Heart of Public Services*. London: Department of Health.

32. National primary care research and development centre (2007) National evaluation of the Expert Patients Programmeme. Available at; http://www.expertpatients.co.uk/NationalEvaluationEPP.pdf [accessed 10th July 2008].

33. Department of Health (2005a) *Self Care: A Real Choice: Self care Support a Practical Option*. London: Department of Health.

34. Department of Health (2005b) *Supporting People with Long Term Conditions. An NHS and Self Care Model to Support Local Innovation and Integration*. London: Department of Health.

35. Department of Health (2006) *Our Health, Our Care, Our Say: a New Direction for Community Services*. London: Department of Health.

36. Newbould J., Taylor D., Bury M. (2006) Lay led self-management in chronic illness: a review of the evidence. *Chronic Illness*. 2(4) 249–61.

37. Tattersall R. (2002) The expert patient: a new approach to chronic disease management for the twenty-first century. *Clinical Medicine*. 2(3): 227–9.

38. Griffiths, C., Motlib, J., Azad, A., et al. (2005) Expert Bangladeshi patients? Randomised controlled trial of a lay-led self management programmeme for Bangladeshis with chronic disease. *British Journal of General Practice*. **55**: 520, 831–7.

Chapter 3

Participants views

The core concern of this book is the experience of people with chronic conditions. This chapter focuses on the experience of three people from widely different contexts. This is not a research report rather it is an attempt to ground the coming discussions in the day-to-day experience of people for whom involvement in a self-management course made a difference. The three contributors, previously unknown to the editor, were identified by Angela Donaldson, Arthritis Care's Training Services Manager in Glasgow; Elizabeth Bayliss, Director of Social Action for Health in Tower Hamlets; and Gail Neillings, EPP Coordinator at The Christie Hospital, Manchester. They were each asked to identify someone who had been through a self-management course and for whom it mattered. In the event, Carol McNaughton writes having done the arthritis course, Challenging Arthritis; Christine Cupid from experience of the CDSMC, where the EPP is supported by the PCT; and an anonymous course tutor writes from the EPP pilot at The Christie in Manchester.

Scottish Lowlands

Carol McNaughton lives near Glasgow. Her GP initially told the 12-year old's parents, she just wanted to dodge school. Although few of her joints remain intact, she is full of praise for her care received at Glasgow's Southern General Hospital. After a Challenging Arthritis course, friends and family commented on changes in stature, confidence, and wellbeing. As her disease improved, she trained to become a course tutor. Four years later, she set up a small business through the *New Deal: Back to Work* programme. She is very active in Arthritis Care.

Carol McNaughton writes

Signing up for Challenging Arthritis, I was not at all sure what I would gain, but I was willing to give it a try. I was a bit tentative about even entering the room, but soon there were 18 of us and in 15 minutes, I was hooked. The course was so good that all 18 continued to the end of the 6 weekly sessions. I came out not only with my certificate but also with confidence, more knowledge of my illness, a more positive outlook on my future, and more awareness of my medication and how to approach my medical team. Indeed, my GP's surgery was so taken by the course that they later became involved with supporting several other Challenging Arthritis courses.

The course covered several aspects of self-management; some I already practiced to get through my daily life, but had never realized I was actually doing – goal setting and relaxation techniques to name two. I soon found myself asking more in depth questions and even found a confidence that I was not aware of before. The morale of the participants was boosted from day one, and we all showed great camaraderie with phone numbers being swapped; I am still in touch with several of the participants after all these years.

After this course finished, I was approached by the Arthritis Care Training Services Manager (TSM) to become a trainer for the Challenging Arthritis courses. This was the start of many years presenting the courses all over North Ayrshire – and I loved it. I actually found myself looking forward to the day of the course for 6 whole weeks and only very rarely was I unable to fulfil my part and ask for a stand-in trainer to take my place. I will always be grateful to the TSM who could see the confident outgoing person that I did not know I was.

I have made many new friends through the courses and a volunteer within Arthritis Care where I now have many 'hats' to wear. I could *never* have done this prior to participating in Challenging Arthritis.

After retiring from course tutor tasks due to illness, I was soon hankering for something to do and went to our local Business Enterprise who helped me start up my own Printing and Design Company. I became very busy as I had managed to slip into a much needed niche in the rural area where I live. I could never have done this without my training and independence gained through challenging *my* arthritis.

I now hope to do further training later this year to become part of the Challenging Pain and Challenging Your Condition teams in Scotland. I continue to set myself daily goals to aim for, and in doing so, I hope to help many others along the way.

Tower Hamlets

Christine Cupid, lives in Tower Hamlets. She has 3 children: 24, 17, and 11. She holds a Diploma in Higher Education, a BTEC National Certificate in Business & Finance and at the time of writing is a third year undergraduate business student. Since 2001, her diagnoses have been accumulating: Spondylosis, Sciatica, (Radiculopathy), Arthritis, Depression, and Severe

Anxiety Disorder. Christine delivers self-management courses in the programme organized by Social Action for Health.

Christine E. A. Cupid writes

Before I did the EPP course, my health was awful. I suffered from severe back pain, depression, anxiety, and also panic attacks. The only times I really left my house were to go to the doctor and even that didn't seem to help. I seemed to be stuck in a cycle – taking medication, picking up more medication – and my treatment wasn't going anywhere.

One day, I was waiting in the doctor's surgery, when I noticed a poster for a self-management course. The words 'Chronic Pain' stood out and so I stored the number in my phone and forgot about it. It was only when Chloe, my daughter, was going through my phone that I remembered what it was. She encouraged me to make the call. I just wanted someone to be there to talk to on the other end, but all I got was the answer machine. Frustrated, I hung up, but called back several days later. Again, I got the answer machine – but this time I left a message. A week later, I received a large envelope in the post full of course information and what seemed like lots of paperwork. At that time, I was in no state to process all that information, so ignored it and pushed it out of my mind.

A few months later, I got a call from the EPP co-ordinator at City and Hackney PCT. He told me that I had missed the original course I had been interested in, but would I like to take part in the next one? My state of mind at the time was such that I found phone conversations difficult and just to get rid of him, I said yes.

However, a call did come several months later inviting me to a course that was starting soon. The man on the end of the line was very keen that I attended, and it was clear that he wanted to help. He even offered transport to and from the venue and so, eventually, I gave in. At that time, my mobility was very limited and a constant struggle. Later, I realized that at that point I hadn't left the house properly for 3 months except to go to GP and consultant appointments.

I had half forgotten about it when the day of the course arrived. An ambulance pulled up outside my house and the driver came to the door and told me he was here to take me to John Scotts Health Centre for the EPP course. He too was very patient, and ended up waiting for me while I got ready. I was 20 minutes late, but Hugh was sitting downstairs, waiting for me. If he hadn't been there for me on that day, I know that I would have got back in the ambulance and gone straight back home. He stayed during the session and I was able to see him out the corner of my eye. This was very reassuring–his patience and support helped me conquer some of the fright I was feeling.

Even so, the first two sessions were very difficult. My chronic pain and depression had left me withdrawn and isolated. It was hard to process the things that were going on around me. This meant that I hadn't really registered what the course was about. By the third week, however, I was beginning to feel a change. For the first time in ages, I attempted to put on make-up. Even being able to do small day-to-day things like that feels monumental when you have been unable to do them for so long. I started talking in sessions, too, much to the delight of the course tutors.

On week 4, my daughter mentioned how much happier I seemed. Before, I had been feeling a lot of guilt and shame about my capabilities as a mother. My children had been the ones looking after me, helping me get out of bed in the morning and to get dressed. My week 4 action plan was to talk to my family and so, one evening, I asked my son what he had done that day in school. He could hardly believe it. He was more used to telling his sister about those kinds of things as I was not able to hold conversation for too long. I had once overheard her telling him 'not to bother mum' about it. From then on, he talked to me every evening, and I was so happy to be able to listen.

When we got to week 5, I couldn't wait for the Monday to come around again because I just knew it would make a difference to my life. At that time, I didn't quite know how but I just knew it would change my life.

When you live with something like chronic pain, it is easy to ignore advice from others. At the course people would suggest distraction techniques: 'read a book', 'listen to music'. It was then that I realized I hadn't listened to music or even picked up a newspaper for ages. When I did, it helped. Just being reminded of these things can be useful – we often forget all about them because we become wrapped up in our conditions. By the end of the course, my pain had lessened and I wasn't taking as much medication. What's more, my doctor told me that I looked better.

The one thing I have kept up from the course, even now with my work as a course tutor, is Action Planning. I still action plan all the time and it was in my action plan to become a course tutor. I continually focus on not getting back into that symptom/pain cycle.

Doctors' reaction to me participating on a course? Both my doctor and my consultant are extremely pleased with my coping methods, acceptance of my condition, and the way I am prepared to challenge my condition knowing it is something I may have to live with for the rest of my life.

Today, my family unit is much happier and more settled. EPP came along at the right time as it not only made a significant difference to me but it also has had a knock on effect on my family.

I've seen how far I've come and the progress I've made. My hope is that in my involvement with delivering the programme, I can share my experiences and help and support as many people as possible.

The Christie, Manchester

This tutor, who prefers to remain anonymous, writes of his experience and continuing involvement. His background is managerial. The programme at The Christie continues within the overall management of the chaplain Revd Kevin Dunn.

Course Tutor writes

I was diagnosed with cancer in January 2006. After surgery, medication, and radiotherapy, my initial treatment schedule was completed in July of the same year. Towards the end of my treatment, I received a letter from the EPP team inviting me to attend a course in January of 2007.

The diagnosis and treatment had had a profound impact on my life and had left me feeling very vulnerable. The course quickly motivated me to regain some of the interests I had before diagnosis and to regain some fitness. By the end of the six-week course, I felt that I had made significant progress. As far as fitness was concerned, there were measurable improvements that, of course, motivated me to continue.

Feeling so positive about the course, I volunteered to train as a tutor and on the residential training course met others, also with chronic conditions. I realized that, while patient's problems vary considerably, there are many common factors for people diagnosed with a chronic condition. Since becoming an accredited tutor, I have co-tutored six courses and find the experience extremely rewarding. The initial meeting of any course brings together people with a very varied range and severity of conditions as well as a wide range of emotions. It is impossible to overstate the psychological impact of a diagnosis of a chronic illness – it is not always life threatening, but is inevitably life changing. I believe the EPP course is a great help in assisting group members come to terms with their condition and helps them learn to manage their lives.

It is noticeable that participants gain much from their fellow group members as well as benefiting from the course content. Many have told me that they were very happy and relieved to be able to discuss their problems with people who had similar conditions and experience – in some cases they found it easier than talking about their feelings with close family members who had no experience of chronic conditions.

The course is not suitable or appropriate for everyone – the very confident person who feels in control of their life will gain little from attending (but if they did attend, fellow participants would gain much from their presence). However, for many people who feel deeply worried about their condition, who are unsure of the future and how to respond to their changed circumstances, I feel that the course is very beneficial.

I continue to tutor when called on for two main reasons – the first is that I truly believe in the benefits of the course. The second is more selfish – I get a great deal of personal satisfaction and pleasure in seeing the participants' progress as the course develops and watching their confidence grow and abilities increase.

Editor

It was experiences very much like these that profoundly affected managers and developers in the mid 1990s. We felt an obligation to make such empowerment experiences available to people struggling to manage lives with arthritis and other long-term conditions. Sometimes, we also glimpsed the possibility of more profound societal change. This came home to us when in 1997 we held a conference at Ashford, Kent. The senior people who came were making connections with wider policy considerations that were to become formative.

Chapter 4

Advanced journeys into self-management

Some people who began as participants have made long journeys into the theory and practice of self-management. In this chapter, another trio offers their experience and reflections. Barbara Hogg has been involved since the earliest days of the work in England. Dr. Andy Turner was a researcher before he was a participant, but has developed special insights related to the usefulness of the ideas in mental health. Kathy Hawley was one of the first round of staff recruited into the EPP and has become a noted developer especially of work with young people.

A personal journey

Barbara Hogg

From age seven, life consisted of a succession of medical appointments. Eventually diagnosed with juvenile chronic arthritis (JCA), the journey began. My parents took most of the treatment decisions and I grew up believing that my condition could be managed by taking my tablets and doing what the doctor told me. I never dared to ask questions. Looking back over that period, I recognize that I was within a 'medical model' of care.

Through my 20s and 30s, the JCA progressed to rheumatoid arthritis (RA) damaging many joints and leaving me feeling I had no control over this disease that caused me such pain, my self-esteem was low. In my mid 30s, my left knee joint was deteriorating rapidly and mobility becoming increasingly limited. I was told that I was 'too young' to be considered for a joint replacement. It was so depressing and I had visions of life in a wheelchair.

Somehow I plucked up the courage to ask for a second opinion. That was a turning point. It resulted in a new knee joint, a new lease of life and a new attitude to the management of my RA. By asking for another opinion, I had made things happen. I realized that I was not communicating well with doctors. How many times had I put on a brave face and said 'I'm fine', when asked how I was managing? About this time, I discovered Arthritis Care and read Arthritis News. Understanding more about my arthritis made me feel more confident about managing the disease and that I could play an active role in managing my RA. When I read that Stanford University had developed a self-management course and Arthritis Care was planning to offer it to their members, I knew immediately I wanted to be involved.

In February 1994, I attended the country's second pilot course[1] in Wellingborough. It was striking that the two leaders were like me, people with arthritis. And they were not talking down to us, they were part of the group. They outlined the next 6 weeks and talked about pain management, exercise, relaxation, nutrition, communicating with our medical team and much more. A growing atmosphere of trust allowed us to share many of each other's problems and anxieties. Each week we made a 'contract' with ourselves, to change our behaviour. Exercise is important in RA, but knowing and doing are not the same thing. Now, swimming became a regular activity. Walking became a habit, depending on my pain and energy levels. In many ways I'd been managing my condition for years: there is no choice. However, taking part in the course added to my knowledge and confirmed I was on the right path. Riding high on my newly discovered confidence, I applied for a job and was appointed a Regional Organizer for Arthritis Care.

I was part of the steering committee that began to roll-out Challenging Arthritis. I applied to be trained as one of the initial corps of course leaders along with four other people from the Wellingborough pilot. The first UK Leader Training was held in August 1994 at Coventry University's Hereward College. Kate Lorig, was assisted by Ann Silvester, Arthritis Care's Information Officer (who had trained in Denmark). I was in at the beginning of something that was able to make a huge difference in the lives of people with arthritis.

Discussions between Arthritis Care and Northamptonshire Social Services now engaged the Adult Education Services, and a 3-year collaborative project called Self Management of ARThritis (SMART) was created. SMART was and remains unique in delivering courses through Adult Education with tutors paid the going rate[2]. Kerstin Goulding, the Adult Education Services County Co-ordinator for Work with People with Disabilities, was appointed as Project Manager. Margaret Oakley, an experienced AE tutor with arthritis, was the Project Co-ordinator.

The project team publicized the courses on local radio and talked to all manner of groups. Despite this, take up was disappointingly slow. GPs in particular seemed wary of this new concept of *lay-led* self-management courses. The breakthrough came unexpectedly, when I was featured in the local newspaper, talking about my personal experience. We were learning that participants want to talk to someone with arthritis before they enrolled on the course. Future course enrolments always offered this option.

We held courses in many different community locations. Participants really appreciated having tutors with experience of living with arthritis. Interestingly, the process of doing the course seems to be as important as the content. For many participants, the course was the first time they had shared how coping with pain and stiffness affected their lives. Discovering positive ways of dealing with these problems gave them hope for a better future. Even some of the Coventry University researchers had arthritis.

By the end of the course, participants were always keen to carry on meetings, and Adult Education Services offered further options. Taster days gave participants opportunities to experience new activities and learn new skills. We had identified a large group of people with arthritis with an interest in self-management, and in May 1996, the Arthritis Care Link Group began with around 40 members. This group continues to flourish and is offering its 100 or so members, monthly meetings, exercise in a warm water pool, ten-pin bowling, Tai Chi and sailing. By the end of the SMART project, 25 courses and 2 Gujarati courses had been delivered.

The time spent with our health professionals is very limited, though vital if disease is to be managed as well as possible. Vastly, more time is spent coping with the pressures of day-to-day living.

Using course tutors with arthritis who act as role models, sends a powerful message to the participants. These tutors understand the emotional impact of living with constant pain, and the anxieties and fears about the future. They show participants, by using self-management techniques, that they are more in control of their condition.

SMART was at the beginning of my personal involvement with the programme. In 1997, I retrained for the generic course. This was very similar in format to the arthritis course, but it felt quite different to be with people with such varied health conditions. Nonetheless, participants soon recognized that everyone in the group shared the same day to day problems. In November 2008, I came full circle as a tutor, when I completed a course with Arthritis Care. The Challenging Arthritis Course will be offered in the county once again in 2009.

Endnotes

1 The UK's second; held in Wellingborough.

2 The rate was shared equally between the two leaders in the early years.

The HOPE course

Andy Turner

Introduction

Self-management research into long-term health conditions (LTHCs) spans the fields of health, social, clinical and medical psychosocial research. The reasons are obvious and understandable, given that many LTHCs cause significant physical and psychological morbidity. Yet, as this contribution will demonstrate neither a psychotherapeutic nor a positive psychological understanding, analysis of self-management has been well articulated and developed. The similarity in outcomes and processes between self-management, group psychotherapy and positive psychology suggests that these might prove useful cannons of work with which to inform and improve self-management research and practice.

A meta-analysis of lay-led self-management programmes confirmed small improvements across several outcomes including self-efficacy, cognitive symptom management, exercise, health distress, anxiety, and depression (1). The fact that the lay-led self-management has the potential to reduce anxious and depressed mood is interesting and sometimes overlooked or downplayed in favour of other outcomes. At any one time, around one in six people in the UK will be experiencing a mental health problem, typically depression and/or anxiety. Nearly, one third of GP consultations are related to mental health problems. A recent study showed that over half of primary care patients assessed by the Hospital Anxiety & Depression scale as 'minimally' depressed were prescribed anti-depressant medication (2). Interestingly, older adults and those with co-morbid physical conditions were less likely to be given any treatment (i.e. medication or referral on to specialized psychological/social/psychiatric services). The National Institute for Clinical Excellence (NICE) guidelines for treating the most common episodes of mental health problems (e.g. mild anxiety and depression) recommend that patients should not be prescribed medication 'because the risk-benefit ratio is poor'. Rather, psychological therapies (e.g. self-help/self-management, cognitive behavioural therapy (CBT)) with an established evidence base should be the first treatment option. However, few patients are routinely offered these therapies due to a shortage of trained therapists and this can be frustrating for GPs and patients alike. A recent meta-analysis suggested that antidepressants are only as effective as placebo treatment for treating people with mild to moderate depression (3).

Coventry University's qualitative evaluations of self-management programmes have identified key group processes appreciated by many participants and tutors. These explain in part why participants attending a 6-week,

15-h programme, delivered by tutors with no psychological/therapy training and where specific depression and anxiety management activities are only briefly and superficially explored, can lead to a reduction in psychological distress. In its own right, the presence of others sharing similar experiences can be extremely beneficial for self-management participants, but the group format also offers the opportunity to experience several other therapeutic (curative) factors. In-depth interviews with participants and tutors over the last 10 years have described the presence of Irvin Yalom's (4) psychotherapeutic curative factors (e.g. instillation of hope, imitative learning, universality and cohesiveness, altruism and self-esteem) on self-management programmes and their relationship with improved outcomes.

Instillation of hope and imitative learning

Seeing others cope effectively with a shared illness instills hope which is an important factor for retaining participants in programmes. Positive expectation and anticipation of a programme's benefits has been associated with successful outcomes. Further, when the client and the therapist have the same high expectations of a programme, there is more likely to be a positive outcome. Yalom has argued that these positive expectations should be encouraged by therapists prior to and in the early stages of a programme. Yalom suggests that group programmes present a powerful source of hope because some participants who are successfully coping will be a role-model of hope for the other participants who are coping less well. Applying this learning from psychotherapy to self-management programmes, it can be seen that it is important for tutors to be confident in their own ability *and* the programme they are delivering to help participants improve. It is also important to identify, emphasize and positively reinforce improvements made by participants so as to instill hope in others.

> *That's the really great thing about the course, seeing how people overcame their problems and lived through them ... I got a boost from these people that if things got worse for me that I could cope.*

Challenging Arthritis participant

> *To chat and laugh and exchange worries and hopes has been helpful. I certainly have a more positive outlook.*

Expert Patients Programme (EPP) participant

Universality & cohesiveness

People living with an LTHC can be reluctant to burden family, friends and health care providers, thus heightening a sense of uniqueness, isolation and anxiety about whether their experiences and feelings are normal. Group self-management programmes can address these feelings of uniqueness and are therefore a powerful source of relief. Some participants in Coventry's research actually referred to the self-management programme as group therapy.

> *It was more like a therapy support group … I suppose it's valuable to know that there are other people out there. Yes, I think that's what I enjoyed about it, was the collective experience of the tutors as well the participants. 'Cos the tutors themselves were sufferers, weren't they.*

Challenging Arthritis participant

Yalom has described this phenomenon as universality – ('we are all in the same boat'). Group programmes can also reduce stigmatization and isolation. Cohesiveness provides social support directly. Yalom describes how group cohesiveness is formed when clients share their anxieties and experiences.

> *Well, at the time I was going through a really bad state of depression and a feeling that you're never going to get any better, and the heart attack could happen again … But going there made me realize that everybody else felt the same, you know when we got talking.*

Expert Patients Programme (EPP) participant

Altruism and self-esteem

Coventry's research has shown that tutors derive benefits from delivering self-management programmes through improved self-esteem and a renewed sense of purpose and meaning in life. Coventry's research has also shown that participants benefit from being able to help other group members either by providing informational support/advice through the problem solving activities and/or providing emotional support by demonstrating empathy, understanding and reassurance. Providing help to others can be as beneficial to health and well being as receiving help. Yalom found that depressed patient' self-esteem improved after realizing that their contributions were important and valued by other group members. Information exchange about living and coping with an LTHC is particularly highly valued, especially if it comes from other participants. Participants are often more likely to accept and value help from others whom they perceive to be similar to themselves. Group programmes are unique in offering participants the opportunity to benefit and help others.

Positive psychology

As we have described, the psychotherapeutic curative factors reported by self-management participants create a positive environment within which to express and experience positive psychological states. Martin Seligman is attributed for officially launching 'positive psychology' as a scientific endeavour during his American Psychological Association Presidential Lecture in 1998. However, as many others have noted, applied positive psychology has a research tradition that spans decades. Linley and Joseph (5) point out that many health professionals are already (unknowingly) using positive psychological techniques to help their clients. Positive psychology is interested in the full range of human functioning and has the dual aims of alleviating psychological distress and promoting positive well-being. Self-management research and practice has tended to focus on the former and hardly at all on the latter with the exception of self-efficacy.

One of Coventry's earliest SMP evaluations included a positive affect outcome measure; the Positive and Negative Affect Scale (PANAS). The PANAS contains 20 adjectives to describe positive and negative emotional states. High positive affect refers to a general tendency to experience a 'state of high energy, full concentration and pleasurable engagement'. Interestingly, the positive rather than negative affect subscale showed improvement. The effect size was similar to self-efficacy effect size (0.3). One of Coventry's Ph.D. students (Dr. Lorraine Mcfarland) explored the role positive emotions have among participants attending self-management programmes in helping them cope. Barbara Fredrickson's broaden and build theory (6) suggests that positive emotions broaden an individual's attention, thinking and action, enabling the building of new, creative thought and action pathways (i.e. expanding the individual's coping skills), and the building of personal and social resources.

HOPE

Coventry's research has identified a renewed and increased sense of hopeful thinking as one of the key improvements among participants attending self-management programmes. Three colleagues (MacHattie, Herganrather, Fotiadou) and I recently developed and delivered a health coaching and support programme, *Help to Overcome Problems Effectively* (HOPE), which is underpinned by hope theory and Fredrickson's broaden and build theory. It also explicitly set out to encourage and exploit several of Yalom's curative factors.

HOPE has been defined as a *'cognitive set that is based on a reciprocally-derived sense of successful agency (goal-directed determination) and pathways (planning to meet goals)'* (7). Although hope theory is similar to self-efficacy theory, there are important differences. Whereas, self-efficacy theory focuses on specific goals/behaviours, hope theory recognizes enduring cross-situational goals/behaviours. Also, self-efficacy theory places more emphasis on agency thoughts (confidence/determination), whereas hope theory places equal emphasis on agency thoughts and pathways thoughts (7). HOPE therapy is designed to help clients conceptualize clear goals and produce numerous pathways to achieve those goals. This is done by reframing barriers that might impede goals as challenges to be overcome. Several HOPE therapy-based studies involving older depressed adults in the United States reported an improvement in hope, and, reduced feelings of hopelessness, anxiety, and depression.

HOPE is an innovative approach to self-management because it encourages positive psychological and behavioural changes by fostering positive psychological emotional states and builds on participants' existing strengths and resiliencies, rather than focusing predominantly on skills deficits.

During the introductory session, for example, participants are invited to create a common identity (universality) with other group members by sharing examples of positive and successful coping attempts rather than sharing problems and failures. Another distinct feature of the first session in the HOPE programme is the introduction of the upward spiral of positive emotions and experiences leading to greater well-being, resilience, and coping. This contrasts with the more common approach in other self-management programmes that introduce a discussion of (the symptom cycle) a negative spiral of fear and frustration leading to negative health and well-being. Other positive psychology techniques in the HOPE programme include keeping a gratitude journal (again introduced in the first session), identifying and describing personal strengths, identifying and engaging in activities that provide meaning and purpose and relaxation techniques. All of these techniques are positive psychological interventions in their own right and have a growing research evidence base. Combined in the HOPE programme, they build an extraordinarily positive experience for participants and tutors alike.

Yet another key element of the HOPE programme, shared with other self-management programmes, is a weekly goal-setting activity. Having goals and sharing them with other participants promotes positive emotional states and successful coping. Goal setting fosters a sense of pride and achievement and participants are inspired and instilled with hope when witnessing others work towards achieving their goals. The HOPE programme emphasizes the importance of *having* goals and *working towards* goals as well as the *completion* of goals. Smail (8) has described the challenges associated with initiating behaviour change and concludes that in many cases there is no alternative to simply '*walking the plank*' of change, which he goes on to stress is less challenging in the presence of encouragement from others. He believes that it is axiomatic that '*doing precedes feeling*' and that for someone to feel better they have to change something in their lives. HOPE has been delivered by our research partners in the United States to groups of Black African Caribbean unemployed men living with HIV/AIDS, and to women with chronic conditions in Greece. HOPE has also been piloted among people living with severe mental health problems via Rethink in the UK. Preliminary data from these studies have shown improvements across a range of variables including hope, thus confirming the theoretically expected (i.e. hope theory) treatment effect, life satisfaction, self-esteem, self-efficacy, and depression. Several participants with depression in the UK study moved one category lower (i.e. participants moved from severe depression to moderate depression or from moderate to lower depression) at follow-up. The following quote from one of the HOPE participants captures the benefits of adopting a positive approach to coping with depression and the impact that this had on other family members; thus confirming Fredrickson's 'broaden and build' theory described earlier. The participant was initially resistant to adopting a more positive mindset, but gradually as a result of undertaking some of the positive psychology techniques she came to see the benefits.

> I think I am better at home, and my daughter is starting to pick up that as well and she's sort of encouraging me to sort of pick up in the home. I've been signed off work the last six years and I've had no incentive, no motivation to do anything around the home at all, so it's in a bit of a state to say the least. That's an understatement and I am beginning now to sort of think, oh yeah I'll do that and I do it. Wow, I've done it! It seems so amazing. Yes the focus on the positives sort of frees your mind from all the negative stuff, so you have energy to do something positive.

HOPE participant

People have a habit of ignoring what goes well and instead pay attention to what is not going so well. Psychologists have developed the gratitude activity: a simple technique to shift the emphasis away from the negative and on to the positive things that are happening in our lives. People, who write a gratitude list, report fewer health complaints, feel more attentive, energetic, determined, more satisfied with life, more optimistic and feel more connected and closer to others. They are also more likely to give help and support to others thereby building social networks and friendships. Below is a quote from one of the HOPE participants describing the benefits of keeping a gratitude list:

> I found it very useful. On the days that you think are disasters, generally there's something hidden away in there that was actually quite good … it might be hard finding it … you don't realize that actually yeah that was actually okay, yeah I managed that, oh, that's another good thing, oh. So it snowballs. It's excellent; it really is a good idea.

HOPE participant

Conclusion

Hope springs eternal

The Department of Health has set out plans to invest £170 million in providing access to individual CBTs through its Improving Access to Psychological Therapies (IAPT) programme. Some have argued that the narrow focus on providing CBT, largely via one-to-one and/or computerized interventions, is short sighted and that the role of mutually supportive self-help interventions delivered via the voluntary sector should be explored (9). There is encouraging work already being undertaken in Australia and the UK involving mental health service users. In Australia, research has shown that patients with a range of severe mental health conditions including schizophrenia found a version of the Chronic Disease Self-Management Course to be helpful. In the UK, the EPP–CIC has developed a self-management programme for people with mental health problems (*New Beginnings*) and a self-management programme incorporating CBT techniques in the Co-Creating Health initiative (see Chapters 12 and 13). Coventry's HOPE programme has produced some encouraging early results. Given the inappropriate prescription of antidepressant medication (3) for patients with mild/moderate depression and inequalities in treatment for depression among elderly patients and patients with LTHCs (2), the focus of this work is clearly warranted.

There is growing interest in applied positive psychology promoting research and practice into factors that enable individuals, communities and societies to flourish and achieve optimal functioning. Fredrickson has shown that positive emotions are an important aspect of flourishing. Hopefully, I have shown here how a combination of Yalom's curative factors, goal setting and the fostering of positive emotions may be the mechanisms through which anxiety and depression are reduced and flourishing enhanced.

Albert Bandura suggests that psychosocial programmes should be evaluated, not only in terms of their effectiveness but also in terms of their social utility. This approach is consistent with the view that a function of self-management programmes is to impact on broader determinants of quality of life (e.g. social participation) rather than narrowly defined clinical outcomes. Only 1 study identified by Foster et al. 2007 systematic review, employed social outcomes (e.g. social connectedness) to evaluate self-management programmes and few used mental health measures such as depression, anxiety, and health distress and even fewer used positive psychological measures. A greater emphasis on social processes and outcomes in self-management is warranted. From our own preliminary HOPE research we would like to see added to this an expanded focus on the role of Yalom's curative factors, positive emotions and positive psychological techniques for building psychological resiliencies and social resources as well as alleviating psychological distress.

The theory, philosophy, and process of developing the Staying Positive Programme for adolescents with long term medical conditions

Kathy Hawley

'Give me the child until the age of seven and I will show you the man.'

Justification of Self-Management Programmes for children

The Jesuits famously said, give me a child at the age of seven and he is mine for life; I would re-interpret this as give me a child at the age of 12 and he could be a good self-manager for life. It has always surprised me that major conferences on self-management generally disregard or demote the issue of children with chronic conditions to a minor position, but concentrate on the issues for adults[1]. This is in the context that major chronic conditions requiring the most assiduous application of self-management are usually diagnosed in childhood like type 1 diabetes, epilepsy, asthma, cerebral palsy, sickle cell, muscular dystrophy, haemophilia, juvenile arthritis, and perinatal acquired HIV. With the advent of more sophisticated scanning technology, there is an increasing awareness of the incidence and earlier diagnosis of Multiple Sclerosis in teenagers[2]. It seems that the starting place for programmes on self-management should therefore be with children. I have chosen the age of 12, based on statistical medical evidence and psychosocial behaviour theory on children's development[3].

The child population in the United Kingdom is in the region of 11.7 million[4]. The incidence of G.P. diagnosed asthma in children is 1.1 million; approximately 180,000 children have type 1 diabetes and approximately 165,000 children are born with cerebral palsy[5]. Add the figures for the incidence of other chronic conditions such as cystic fibrosis, epilepsy, sickle cell anaemia, spina bifida, Crohn's disease, juvenile arthritis, haemophilia, and HIV conditions to these statistics, and the scale of chronic disease in children becomes much clearer. Allowing for the fact that some children may have more than one diagnosed chronic condition, the percentage incidence is in the region of 15–17%, which closely aligns with that of the United States where 18% is the accepted figure. These figures emphasize the reality of the scale of chronic disease in children and young people.

All chronic conditions have one thing in common which is, poor self-management of the condition leads to increased demands on the health, social and education services with rises in morbidity and mortality. A good example of this phenomenon is Asthma, where every 18 min a child is admitted to hospital in the U.K.[6]. Most of these admissions are preventable by the use of appropriate good self-management. At a local level, a primary care trust with a population of 100,000, can expect 4,000 children to have a diagnosis of asthma with approximately 60 emergency admissions per year[7]. The peak time for decline in self-management skills is in early adolescence, and theories of child development provide the explanation for this trend[8]. It is the period when young people begin to reject adult supervision in an attempt to establish their own independence and align themselves with their peer groups. At the same time, research shows that once problems of self-management become established, they become difficult to rectify.

The Cochrane Data Base provides detailed examples of projects evaluating the outcomes of using self-management programmes for adolescents with chronic conditions[9]. These uniformly confirm some of the positive effects such as reductions in emergency hospitalizations, reductions in the number of school days lost and the improved psychosocial well-being of the young people. It is therefore logical that there are universal benefits in the use of self-management programmes for young people with chronic conditions.

Forms of self-management for children and adolescents

Self-management techniques can be acquired in a variety of ways, and there are many examples of successful small projects throughout the U.K. One such example is activity holidays organized by Asthma UK. Other programmes use specifically designed projects involving attendance on a weekly basis over a period of time as, for example, the SHINE Project in Sheffield for Childhood Obesity. Another approach involves the use of interactive adventure video games by hospital departments, which subtly teach self-management skills[10]. There are several drawbacks to most of these projects. Some are very costly to run and thereby limited to a small number of children. Many are disease-specific, thereby reinforcing the medical model which leaves young people seeing themselves as a 'disease' and not as a normal teenager. Some isolate (as in the video games) the teenagers from their peers, reinforcing a major problem which young people themselves highlight, that of social isolation.

The children's pilot

After the introduction of the Expert Patients Programme in the U.K., many health care professionals expressed interest in developing the programme for teenagers. The initial Children's Pilot in 2004, which aimed to do this, found that the format of the Lorig model of the Chronic Disease Self-Management course being delivered throughout the NHS was not consistent with the needs or wants of the age group. Further consultation and research with adolescents established that some of the course contents matched up with the issues they had highlighted, but there were many more additional issues which the Lorig model did not include or address[11]. Further research and consultations with the young people established that one-day workshops, which included a fun element as well as the issues on self-management, were their preferred choice for delivery. To this end, I devised a workshop and trialled it in Oxford with a group of 10 young participants with a range of chronic conditions. Two trained young facilitators delivered the workshop. The feedback from all involved on which parts of the workshop were success-ful and what changes would need to be made enabled me to write *The Staying Positive* programme. Eight national sites were established to pilot the new programme, and from these, young facilitators were recruited and trained to deliver the workshops to their peers. Feedback was ongoing from these sites and where essential, adaptations were made to the workshop contents.

Oxford University Department of Primary Health Care was commissioned to undertake an external evaluation, which was completed in October 2007[12]. Some of the key findings included the following:

♦ Young people thought that the Workshops provided new perspectives and ways of thinking about dealing with the difficulties they faced in their daily lives.

♦ All young people interviewed indicated that having young facilitators who also have a chronic condition was a key factor in achieving the aims of the workshop programme.

♦ The workshops helped the young people to become aware of the impor-tance of self care and the consequences of poor management.

♦ The workshops underlined the importance of medication adherence and participants made changes in this area of self-management.

♦ Workshops helped young people to understand the importance of talking to doctors directly rather than relying on their parents.

♦ Many young people reported learning new ways to communicate with doctors and nurses.

♦ The workshops were useful for discussing difficulties at school and provided some ideas for improving school life.

Participants put forward ideas on improving the workshop contents. One such example was the inclusion of an activity on sibling relationships. The need for this, once raised by participants, became obvious. My search for information on the issues faced by young people with chronic conditions drew a blank. All the research work done has concentrated on the issues and problems faced by the healthy siblings. Feedback from participants indicated they had major issues to contend with in how they were perceived and treated by their siblings. For example, they have to deal with the guilt arising from parental focus on them, which detracts from the attention their siblings might otherwise have had. In addition, young people with chronic conditions were often treated as immature or the baby in the family who needs protecting despite the fact that managing a condition at an early age accelerates your level of maturity.

Lessons learnt from the pilot stage

Albert Bandura's theory of Self-Efficacy is a major concept applied to adult self-management programmes to explain why they are effective. This theory, in the very early stages of the pilot, was very much to the forefront. It became abundantly clear as the pilot progressed that lack of ability or capabilities was not something which could be said of many of the participants. In a filming session, for a promotional DVD for the *Staying Positive Programme,* two young lads with type 1 diabetes explained the daily management of their condition; monitoring their blood sugars, measuring their food intake, and calculating the amount of insulin needed for their injections. They had an array of equipment displayed on a table as they talked through its uses and application.

This manifestation of competency in managing the daily requisites of a long-term condition appeared frequently in the workshops. So, it became necessary to analyse other theories to explain the decline in self-management in the adolescent years, when it was clear that the young people were competent to carry out the tasks. The first activity in the workshop is about distinguishing issues that arise from being a teenager and those that arise from having a condition. As the other activities were delivered, it became obvious what the real key was in self-management problems for teenagers. The need to be a normal teenager took precedence over the need to self-manage. Fitting in with your peers is paramount and this accorded with Erikson's theory of child development[13]. Once I acknowledged this, I understood why the rest of the workshop contents worked since they were all placed in managing your condition in the context of peer relationships. So, a major move had been made from the theory of Self-Efficacy to the theory of Normalization. Recent research by others reinforces my own conclusions about the role self-efficacy plays versus Normalization Theory in the context of adolescent chronic disease[14].

Post-pilot problems in the delivery of the *Staying Positive* programme

It was clear from the success of the pilot that the programme had much to offer young people living with a long-term medical condition, and the DH decided that it should become more widely available. This brought new challenges in terms of getting it to a wider audience at a time when the arrangements for delivery would change. At the end of the pilot stage, the Department of Health transferred the *Expert Patients Programme* into a Community Interest Company (EPP–CIC). The new CIC was expected to raise its income from commissions for its services which implied that, as well as dealing with the logistics of mainstreaming a new service, project staff had to market the service to potential purchasers.

In order to take away some of the pressure generated by the need to obtain commissions and allow for the expansion of the workshops in areas of greatest opportunity as well as those where commissions could be secured, I successfully applied for the Vinvolved Grant. This allowed the programme to continue to develop independently of commissions through the appointment of a project manager to oversee its rollout; the finances to train young facilitators and the finances to cover the costs of the workshops. The CIC was very successful in obtaining commissions which together with the V Grant and investment from the CIC meant the programme could potentially expand quite quickly, but delivery to time tables influenced by the commissions in particular have posed problems. The main difficulty has been recruitment of participants. Much time has been spent analyzing the reasons for this, and many of the obvious issues affecting recruitment such as effective marketing and focused use of staff-deployment time have been addressed. The programme also clearly has an appeal to those who attend since the external evaluation had shown that young people had genuinely enjoyed and benefited from the workshops. I concluded, therefore, that a crucial cause of non-recruitment to the workshops must have a more deep rooted cause and may be one which little research has addressed namely self-perception of chronic disease in adolescents.

Self-perception of chronic disease and its relationship to recruitment

Adolescents are a notoriously reluctant to get engaged in certain kinds of projects and the *Staying Positive Programme* was no exception in the early stages. One of the elements of successful recruitment at the pilot stage depended extensively on the personal knowledge by the health care professional of the individual young people. This was a crucial factor in the development of the work and is something I called Cor et Anima: the Heart and Soul. The heart and soul demands that you understand chronic disease primarily from the perspective of the patient/adolescent. The professional perspective must take secondary place.

Self-perception of chronic disease fits into the theory of normalization, in which many young people see their condition as a stigma[15]. They will consider the costs of identifying themselves as having a disability in the context of then having to deal with the said social stigma and discrimination. Thus, if your peer groups are not aware of your stigma, then you will fit in more easily as a normal teenager. This may be one of the explanations why teenagers are reluctant to become involved in workshops. Where their conditions are not obvious, for example, sickle cell, children with invisible conditions may try to avoid the needed health maintenance in an effort to be normal[16]. Professor Marjorie Olney from San Diego University has done several research projects to look at this aspect of disability and chronic disease and her findings correlate with my arguments on reluctance to reveal your condition other than to very close and trusted friends.

Conclusions

Based on the outcomes of the external evaluation of the Staying Positive Programme and on the continuous feedback from young participants, the aims of improving self-management with accompanying psychosocial well-being in adolescents of chronic conditions can be achieved. The areas which led to initial problems in recruitment to the Staying Positive programme, are all remediable at this stage with a possible exception. This exception is around the concept of self-perception of chronic disease by adolescents. It is an area which has been grossly under researched, and which I will address with my research colleagues[17].

Endnotes

1 For example Conference Harrogate 2009 *Managing Long Term Conditions.*

2 Paediatric Multiple Sclerosis: A Report from an M. S Workshop, January 2008.

3 See Erik Erikson's Fifth Stage of Social-Emotional Development in Children and Teenagers.

4 2001 Census.

5 Statistics based on calculations reported by the leading Children's Health Charities.

6 Asthma U.K.

7 Key Facts and Statistics: Asthma U.K.

8 See footnote 3.

9   The University of Manchester School of Nursing are currently undertaking a mapping and evaluation of self care programmes in England.

10   *Packy and Marlon* is a game used by the Kaiser Permante Clinic for children with diabetes.

11   Hawley K. Report on the Children's Pilot. EPP/CIC, 2005.

12   Salinas ME. Evaluation of the Staying Positive Programme. Department of Primary Health Care University of Oxford; October 2007.

13   See Erikson's Theories of Child Development.

14   Antle BJ. Seeking strengths in young people with physical disabilities: learning from the self-perceptions of children and young adults, 2000.

15   Quote from 17 year old with Sickle Cell.

16   Evans T. A Multidimensional Assessment of Children with Chronic Physical Conditions. Health and Social Work, August 2004.

17   See the many papers written by Professor Annette La Greca, University of Miami.

References

1.   Foster G, Taylor SJC, Eldridge SE, Ramsay J, Griffiths CJ. (2007) Self-management education programmes by lay leaders for people with chronic conditions. *The Cochrane Database of Systematic Reviews*. Issue 4. Art. No.: CD005108. DOI: 10.1002/14651858. CD005108.pub2.

2.   Tony K., Christopher D., Anita M., et al. (2009) Management of depression in UK general practice in relation to scores on depression severity questionnaires: analysis of medical record data. *British Medical Journal*. **338**: b750.

3.   Kirsch I, Deacon BJ, Huedo-Medina TB., et al. (2008) Initial severity and antidepressant benefits: a meta-analysis of data submitted to the food and drug administration. *PLoS Med*. **5**(2): e45 doi:10.1371/journal.pmed.0050045.

4.   *Yalom ID., Leszcz M. (2005) *Theory and Practice of Group Psychotherapy* (5th Edition). New York: Basic Books.

5.   *Linley PA., Joseph S. (editors) (2004) *Positive Psychology in Practice*. New York: Wiley.

6.   Fredrickson B.L. (1998) What good are positive emotions? *Review of General Psychology*. **2**: 300–19.

7.   *Snyder (2000) *Handbook of Hope Theory, Measures and Applications*. California: Academic.

8.   Smail D. (1996) *How to Survive Without psychotherapy*. London: Constable.

9.   Gilbert P. (2009) Moving beyond cognitive therapy. *The Psychologist*. **22**: 400–01.
     *Books recommended for further reading

Chapter 5

The principles of lay leadership

Jean Thompson MBE

Ethos of lay-led self-management

The first lay-led self-management course in the UK was the Arthritis Self-Management Course (ASMC) developed at Arthritis Care. The opportunity to progress this pioneering work was provided by Richard Gutch (RG), CEO who created the space for a UK-wide programme to be developed. He initially had to contend with scepticism within and without the organization, as it was generally a time of financial austerity. Many reservations were overcome as time went on and self-management courses were seen to provide a toolkit for people to use daily to stay in control as much as possible in order to be 'fully engaged with their lives' (Wanless)[1].

ASMC course participants demonstrated their new found confidence to manage their condition by taking on new challenges, as the course often had a ripple effect into other parts of their lives. Many participants sought training to become tutors and they often became amongst the most committed and passionate. They were the best advocates and became more engaged with living their own lives as fully as possible, being seen as excellent role models that often convinced the sceptics about the power of the approach.

People, organization, and politics

The driving force for me in developing lay-led self-management programmes was that they could provide an opportunity, not only for people with a long-term condition (LTC) to gain important skills but also to experience powerful feelings of personal worth, dignity, and validation through facilitating others to make changes.

I place much emphasis on the need for programmes where appropriate to be 'Lay Led'. It underlines the fact that people living with a LTC, are often in the best position to understand how it can be managed with the support of, rather than the control of, health care workers. It could be summed up by the phrase 'nothing about us without us'. (See Bob Sang's work[2])

Involvement in this pioneering work was immensely exciting: Arthritis Care had a special role as an initiator of lay-led self-management courses and later, cooperation with other user-governed organizations through the Long-term Medical Conditions Alliance (LMCA) ensured that course availability was extended to other patient groups. The decision by RG that the next CEO should preferably be someone with arthritis was of profound symbolic importance to people with arthritis involved in the programme. We struggled to convince the Medical Advisory Committee of the significance of lay-led self-management and although at this time there were opportunities for those of us who saw the importance of the self-management to seize power positions in the organization, we failed to recognize or seek these opportunities. The fact is we shared a service delivery motivation. That was our main preoccupation and priority and, probably quite wrongly, we trusted others to ensure we had the space to operate in.

A turning point came when it was agreed to send me to Stanford for Master Trainer training for the generic course, the Chronic Disease Self-Management Course (CDSMC). In the UK, we had realized early on that multiple co-morbidity was a feature of the course participants in Challenging Arthritis (CA). As a result of this training, I became an important resource for extending the capability of Arthritis Care to deliver a generic self-management course even though the organization was reluctant to look at extending its mission beyond people with arthritis. It was keen to share values and expertise, however, and develop capacity in other organizations. Thus, a trading arm was established through which Arthritis Care offered training and consultancy to other patient organizations to establish their own quality assured self-management programmes.

New central service development management, for example, did not appear to understand the potential national policy significance of what was being done and often seemed to see self-management as just a course with marketing potential. Critical support was therefore lost for key aspects of the value system shared by myself, Roy Jones (RJ), and Keith Hawley (KH) the three consultants operating within the trading arm at a time when regional directors had assumed greater power and influence seeming bent on diluting the power of the centre. The effect was that Arthritis Cares leadership in lay-led self-management stalled. Key people who had earned the credibility to influence national policy and explain the values of role modelling and empowerment of people with LTCs felt sidelined.

With the publication of the white paper, *Saving Lives, Helping People* came a task force, involving statutory and voluntary sector leaders to develop the idea of the Expert Patient. Its report was published in 2001 and a pilot scheme began. The Department of Health (DH) could have involved the voluntary sector more, but it was still a triumph for ideas originating in Arthritis Care.

The work done by KH with local social services departments, encouraging them to see lay-led self-management programmes as supportive to independence strategies, seemed to fall into abeyance. RJ whose inspiration and networking had been such an asset and source of resources was made redundant and there was a major loss of morale amongst the actual deliverers. Richard who had created space for the programme left, as did eventually the rest of the original trio, dispirited and frustrated. It was generally a most unhappy time for many who had worked hard at all levels to create a very exciting, successful, and life changing programme built on passion for changing the lives of people with an LTC through partnership working and freely sharing ideas, experiences, and expertise. A programme that had captured the imagination of academics, patient bodies, professionals, and the funding of Government seemed to squander its potential at the very point at which that had been recognized.

Reflection

It is not clear whether the problems in Arthritis Care (AC) were personality or structurally based. In voluntary sector agencies, it is often services that go down in financial hard times.

LMCA

(later Long Term Conditions Alliance and now absorbed into National Voices)

We developed a useful training resource and considerable experience in developing quality assured lay-led programmes which was useful to support organizations in LMCA to build capacity as deliverers. LMCA gained funding from the Royal College of Physicians to support member organizations develop self-management programmes. It was a pivotal moment when we convinced them to use the CDSMC in the first instance, rather than waste time trying to write a new course and attempt to secure some consensus from the medical profession as to what should go in it! The self-management programme at LMCA started with Living with Long-term Illness (Lill) managed by Jane Cooper (JC).

Reflection

JC enjoyed what was denied to us in Arthritis Care. She was fully supported to market and celebrate the Lill project. Despite the small number of tutors and courses involved, it had enormous impact.

The internal structures and stresses that emerged in Arthritis Care meant it gradually took away the resources to market and advertise the considerable achievements including the leadership role, UK coverage and size of programme. In consequence, the programme stalled.

Humanitarian values

Self-management is not something you give to people nor is it optional for people who have a LTC. A person with an LTC has no choice but to self-manage but they can choose to do it actively or passively. The courses are about moving a person to action, facilitating the building of confidence in achieving small steps to improve daily life. The course participants operate as support groups for the six weeks. In that time, individuals regain their 'helper roles' that have often been taken away due to people in their lives 'helping' them too much.

Self-management training is about sharing; not about having a body of knowledge poured in. People appropriate and use the courses according to their needs, but there is a key underlying assumption, namely that participants and tutors alike are all trying to live as full a life as possible despite their LTC. They are about minimising the impact of chronic disease(s).

The people who gain most from these courses are able to communicate more effectively with family, doctors, and health professionals and are confident that they can manage life with their condition(s) making day-to-day use of their developing problem solving skills. But confidence is often fragile. It is crucial, therefore, that all are supported to make changes by health care professional teams, and the NHS system supports both patients and staff to engage in mutually respectful relationships, recognizing one another's expertise.

This is the way resources in communities need to be built. If communities are going to fully engage, they need to be supported and maintained through a lay-led approach.

Personal reflection

When I went to Arthritis Care, the time was right for ASMC known by us as CA. CA was a success when people with a passion for it were in the driving seat. The organization at that time had identified a need to support people with arthritis fulfil their life roles, regain confidence lost, find themselves again, activate their inner resources, and not be an 'arthritic'. Actively recruiting people with arthritis to be deliverers, in addition to fulfilling key managerial roles, meant we attracted some very resourceful special people who added to the richness of the programme.

I had come from education and therefore tackled the recruitment and training as 'life-long learning' and self-management as 'life-long health' I could lead the programme as I had earned the right to do so due to my experience of life and living with a LTC. My education and training qualified me to fulfil the role. I could recruit, manage, and lead a team of people with LTCs as I role modelled this approach throughout my practice. The organization provided the right base in which to achieve success and for the first time I felt 'I had come home'. All my life's experiences proved useful in developing programmes.

The meeting of AC and LMCA came at the right time just after I returned from the CDSMC training in Stanford. In addition, I always think it is about relationships. I think Roy, Keith, and I all had the right skills as a team and I, with my team of people with LTCs, respected Richard's approach. This meant we worked our socks off for little financial reward to make it happen in AC. Psychologically and physically, it came at the right time as previously I had avoided people with arthritis; my flare ups were becoming far less eventful and debilitating, I had ended an emotionally abusive relationship, my boys were in their teens and my dad had moved in, providing after school care. All of these things were crucial in allowing me to travel the breadth and depth of the UK (later other continents) recruiting, training marketing, and role modelling the approach and building capacity.

The DH approach to the pilot EPP was fundamentally flawed as they set up a costly infrastructure, falling into the trap of thinking about the courses rather than the sustainability of a programme. Initially, there were no real resources put into changing the organizational approach of the NHS or training of health care professionals to enable them to engage differently with people with LTCs.

We could not have gained some of the many benefits that have been achieved despite the above caveats without key supporters such as Ayesha Dost in the DH and the Chief Medical Officer of Health's input. We have reached communities that were previously not included. A unique workforce was created both prior to EPP in the voluntary sector and then with in EPP. A workforce of people with LTC for people with LTC. The single most disappointing outcome is that this unique approach is being corroded by a business model. When EPP was first created, it was almost unique as it had been in the voluntary sector, driven by and for people with LTCs providing a real learning curve for DH.

We have achieved so much in EPP and put self-management on the map. But to achieve choice and world class commissioning there now needs a fundamental shift back to the Living with Lill project days of supporting a wide variety of organizations to become providers ensuring all communities benefit.

Endnotes

1 Wanless D. 'Securing our future health; taking a long term view' (Final report).

2 Sang B. 'Health gain, the true test of quality for 21st century healthcare'.

Chapter 6

Delivering courses now

Programmes delivering self-management courses have been launched in many contexts. This chapter looks at a few. These are important examples, but understate the variety and subtlety of many local initiatives. Here, we have contributions from the English and the Scottish experience, the development of the online (English) version, working within Tower Hamlets Bengali communities and the background effort to establish consensus and a Quality Institute.

Looking at the Expert Patients Programme

Jim Phillips

The 2006 White Paper, *Our Health, Our Say, Our Care* (1) set out a commitment to expand and diversify the EPP. Programmes were to be designed and delivered in way that increased the diversity of people attending by the development of:

- Disease-specific courses
- Courses relevant to specific communities
- Multiple modes of delivery

In response, the EPP–CIC has expanded its programme to include:

- Courses in 9 languages
- Courses in all the main disease types and developing programmes in the remaining gaps
- Developing or considering a range of delivery modes. For example, in groups, on-line, and by distance learning
- Meeting longer term support issues through post-course support groups, networks and online communities
- A range of evidenced based materials aimed at people at risk of developing a long-term condition (LTC) and at improving general self care of lifestyle risks areas – diet, exercise, and emotional well-being.

However, the current NHS commissioning model is too narrow to fully meet the needs of people with LTCs and has shifted the emphasis on the role of the programmes.

It is worth looking at some of the original motivating factors for lay-led self-management. In 2001, the department of health commissioned a set of focus groups to gain the views of the public on self care. One of the questions asked to the participants was how do they rate the level of support they receive from their health care team? The majority of participants regardless of age, condition, etc. all reported that while they rated the actual contact with a clinician highly, they all felt that there was a lack of support for dealing with the *impact* of their health condition on their daily lives.

It is this gap in support that lay-led self-management programmes were designed to fill and links back to the main principle in developing such programmes, namely the question 'what do you want, as a person with a long-term health condition, to be able to improve your life?'– It was this that made EPP so popular with participants and voluntary organizations. Lay-led self-management provided a means by which people could improve their quality of life and deal with the consequences of their health condition.

With the publication of the Wanless report and the setting up of the EPP, we have seen a shift in emphasis of what is expected from self-management programmes. There has been a move away from seeing quality of life, self-determination, and coping strategies as important and justifiable outcomes in their own right, and the main driving factor, to a focus on health service utilization and savings to the NHS. This shift from being *patient led* back to being *service led* has subtly distorted the original purposes. For lay-led self-management and the EPP to be a long-term, financially sustainable part of patient care, models of delivery need to take into account both the support needs of the patient and the outcomes sought by service commissioners. In other words, the needs of the patient must be paramount in the commissioning of self-management services.

Current models of EPP provision fit into two broad categories:

Those delivered by an organization as part of its services.

This is the one most associated with voluntary organizations such as Arthritis Care, Body Positive (North West), etc. Here, we see good utilization of volunteers, generally supported by a staff member who is also able to train and support them. Some PCTs also deliver their services in this way with a coordinator running several patient support programmes. Organizations are generally able to run their self-management programmes at relatively low cost, around £200 per person. The model may include the provision of some commissioned programmes. Key advantages of this model are the low cost and ability to easily signpost participants to other more specialized support such as help with housing, welfare benefits, etc. that these organizations also provide.

Stand-alone commissioned programmes.

This is where Primary Care Trusts directly commission the provision of blocks of course places usually by 100. These have largely been driven by PCT tenders that ask for courses to be provided in the community, but with no tie-in to other services such as diabetes or asthma care, etc. This approach by PCTs leads to poor targeting of resources, difficulties in recruitment, and inappropriate referral. It is difficult in these circumstances to maximize the benefits of self-management peer learning to the wider system.

(a) The way forward

There is an a priori need to move towards an integrated self care pathway. This requires greater integration with health care services and an improvement in the current commissioning model so that the best elements of the locally delivered programmes are included and secured. Similarly, there needs to be a shift of delivery to local providers who can ensure that a network of support services can be linked to the programmes providing a much stronger connection with clinical and social care services. In order to achieve these possibilities, the key role of local coordinator, identified in both voluntary sector forerunners and early pilots, needs to be established. It personalizes support for enquirers and volunteers, as well as managing and maintaining local networks, within formal services and reaching into local communities.

Evidence from the RCT shows that some people benefit more than others from the programmes (2). Where provision is part of the NHS service and resources are restricted it would make sense to ensure that those who are in greatest need and would benefit the most should be targeted. In addition, to ensure that the two core outcomes criteria are met – cost effectiveness and quality of life – it is important that this becomes an integrated case-managed service.

(b) Who should be targeted?

Evidence suggests that those who stand to benefit the most are people:

With low quality of life

Having difficulty in changing lifestyle

With low self-confidence

Who have already received basic health education about their condition.

It should be relatively straightforward for a PCT or GP surgery to identify a clear cohort of people who could be referred to self-management support.

Some points from the Darzi report (3):

The report has brought forward other points relevant to taking forward self-management. Inter alia it proposes:

- Individual care plans for all people with LTCs
- Introduction of personalized budgets
- Access to healthy living services to support control of alcohol use, exercise, etc.
- A patient prospectus to provide advice on how to manage LTCs
- Integrated community-based services
- Support for people to stay healthy at work and return to work
- World class commissioning with strong emphasis on patient involvement and individually tailored care

Responding to these considerations would lead to the construction of a whole pathway approach to self care that would offer individualized care packages tied in to individual care plans (Fig. 6.1).

Such a model would provide better integration with health and social care services. It is here that the tangible benefits of these programmes would be, and in some places are, already experienced. These are predominately

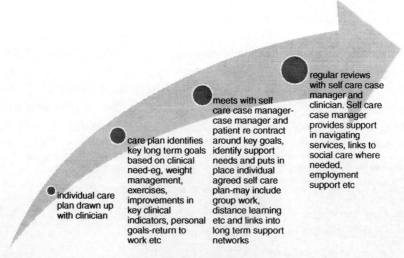

Fig. 6.1 Securing self-care in the Individual Care Plan.

in the reduction of GP and nurse time in dealing with related health issues. In addition, the case manager would be in a position to act as a support for individual budget holders.

Patient support needs would be fully assessed ensuring those of highest need are fully supported and linked to the most appropriate services.

(c) And, not finally

The centrality of the patient, being the prime actor in the care of people with a long-term health condition, needs to be re-established. Only when people have a substantial sense of control do they discover what they are capable of. There is good reason to think current models too often engender dependency on service providers. The potential for self care among people with LTCs has been demonstrated, now the structures need to adapt for a more active partnership between people and their health and social care professionals.

The programme in Scotland

Angela Donaldson

Policy Background

The Scottish Parliament was established in 1999 following a referendum by the Labour Westminster government of the Scottish people, where 74% of voters were in favour. Scots feelings of discontent with Westminster developed during the Thatcher years, and people did not feel appropriately represented by a Conservative government at Westminster. The Scotland Act, which legislated for the establishment of the Parliament, also gave it sole responsibility for the development of health policy in Scotland.

Constitutionally, the Parliament established mechanisms for public involvement across every area of responsibility, and a 'compact' was developed with the Voluntary Sector to ensure their involvement at all appropriate levels. Although these mechanisms have worked with varying degrees of effectiveness, the commitment to finding more and better ways of supporting the processes has been a priority for the Parliament itself.

Challenging Arthritis – Stanford University model in Scotland

The Challenging Arthritis course was introduced into Scotland by Arthritis Care in 1994 as part of a 3-year project funded by the Scottish National Lotteries Charity Board (SNLCB). This enabled the infrastructure to be developed to deliver the programme, with highly trained and well-supported volunteers, in a variety of locations across the country. With the cessation of the SNLCB funding, the development of Challenging Arthritis in Scotland was for the next few years, dependent on charitable donations and small grants from local authorities or health boards. A lack of awareness of self-management as a concept meant that development was patchy at this time.

Promoting the concept of lay-led self-management and its benefits to policy makers and health professionals became a priority for Arthritis Care across the UK with considerable success. However, where the Expert Patient Programme (EPP) was developed with the Department of Health in England, Arthritis Care in Scotland recognized self-management as core to their own direct service delivery, with the potential to influence how services were developed in the statutory sector, as well as providing an income stream for the organization while continuing to promote self-management within the political arena.

In 2002, the Public Health Institute for Scotland led by Professor Phil Hanlon published a Scottish Needs Assessment Report for Rheumatoid Arthritis. Arthritis Care in Scotland represented the patient perspective on this report, and was successful in ensuring that access to lay-led self-management courses were a key recommendation within it.

Shifting the focus of Scotland's health policy

In 2005, the Kerr Report was published after 14 months of investigation into the state of Scotland's health and care services. Many of the recommendations made by Professor David Kerr's group were contained within the Scottish Executive's Delivering for Health framework, which introduced measures to change the focus of NHS Scotland towards:

◆ Geared towards LTCs

◆ Embedded in communities

◆ Team-based

◆ Continuous care

◆ Integrated care

◆ Preventative care

◆ Patient as partner

◆ Self care encouraged and facilitated

◆ Carers supported as partners

◆ High Tech

Self-management was recognized as a key part of making the necessary culture shift within the population and the NHS itself to address the issues of Scotland's ageing population. They were faced with the increased prevalence of LTCs among people receiving inadequate support and coping with wider social, economic and health inequalities.

Developing voluntary sector capacity – the Long-Term Conditions Alliance Scotland

One of the key recommendations of the Kerr Report was that a Long-Term Conditions Alliance be established, to bring together the voluntary sector voice and provide a focus for the issues shared across all LTCs, including self-management. The Long-Term Conditions Alliance Scotland (LTCAS) was launched in May 2006 with a Board and constitution ensuring that conditions such as arthritis, diabetes, epilepsy, and cancer were represented, alongside young people, carers, smaller community groups, and rarer conditions. The alliance also developed an associate membership for professional groups, but without the same voting rights as the voluntary sector membership.

Developing self-management for LTC

Given the shifting focus of health policy towards the management of LTC in 2004, Arthritis Care in Scotland took the decision to invest in training its self-management teams to offer the Chronic Disease Self-Management courses for people living with all LTCs, in addition to Challenging Arthritis. This programme was particularly useful for Scotland's rural and island communities, where the sparse population meant that courses for specific conditions could neither ensure quality nor cost effectiveness.

Recognizing the need to involve the wider voluntary sector in the development of the self-management agenda, and that their self-management expertise was a potential source of contract income, Arthritis Care in Scotland established an informal group of organizations representing a range of LTCs, with an interest in developing their own self-management programmes. During this period, partnership agreements were developed between AC Scotland and the MS Society Scotland, and Greater Glasgow Health Board, to establish and monitor their own Chronic Disease self-management programmes. In addition, Arthritis Care in Scotland also helped develop programmes in Ireland and Lithuania, with the sister organizations within those countries.

Developing a strategy for managing LTCs in Scotland 'Gaun Yersel'

A large conference was held in November 2006 to promote self-management with policy makers and health professionals. Arthritis Care in Scotland and the MS Society led its organization, recognizing that the event would gain wider support if the newly established LTCAS took ownership of it. The 'Gaun Yersel' event was very successful, with the Scottish Health Minister Andy Kerr MSP as the keynote speaker. Over 200 people attended from all across Scotland; including senior policy makers, health professionals and people with LTCs themselves.

In spring 2007, the Scottish Executive Health Department, took the unprecedented step of asking the LTCA to write the Government's self-management strategy for LTCs in Scotland. Due to be presented to the Executive in the autumn to ensure its inclusion within the budget, the time scales slipped due to the outcome of the Scottish Parliament elections in May 2007, which resulted in a change of leadership in the Parliament: the Scottish National Party formed a minority government. The new Cabinet Secretary for Health and Well-being, Nicola Sturgeon, reaffirmed the Government's support for the self-management agenda within the Better Health, Better Care report, and she earmarked £11million for the LTCAS, with £5 million specifically for developing voluntary sector capacity to deliver self-management.

The LTCAS had established a subgroup, including expertise in self-management, mental health, and homeopathy to develop the self-management strategy for Scotland, and 'Being Human – A Strategy for Managing Long-Term Conditions in Scotland', authored by Susan Douglas-Scott (CEO, Epilepsy Scotland), and myself. It was presented to the Government in January 2008.

The strategy takes a broad view of self-management, and sets out challenges for individuals and organizations around the key stages of a person's journey with an LTC:

- Diagnosis
- Living for today
- Progression
- Transitions
- End of life

Using case studies, the strategy shows how agencies using an approach that supports people to manage their own condition, can help achieve a more positive outcome for people living with one or more LTCs. The 'Scottish model' self-management strategy has also attracted the interest of LTCAs in Northern Ireland and Wales.

Scotland's Self-Management Strategy was launched by Nicola Sturgeon, Cabinet Secretary for Health and Well-being on 4th September 2008, in Edinburgh's Dynamic Earth. The Chief Medical Officer for Scotland, Dr. Harry Burns, has established a self-management sub group at the highest level within the Scottish

Government Health Directorates to progress this agenda, and the LTCA chairs the group.

The Strategy for Managing LTCs in Scotland supports the development of a variety of approaches to supporting self-management, and recognizes the key role of the Stanford University Chronic Disease Programme in improving the current health behaviours of the Scottish population.

The Federation of Small Businesses Index of Success in 2007 showed Scotland in tenth place out of ten for small countries in Western Europe. Scotland performs strongly on educational attainment, which should suggest above average potential for both employment rates and per capita GDP, Scotland's poor overall score is believed mainly attributable to its poor health record.

The Scottish Government appear committed to providing people with support to manage their own LTCs, and regard it as key to addressing some of the wider issues such as health inequality, and the associated social and economic problems of the nation as a whole. 'Gaun Yersel'. We live in hope.

Why we chose to get engaged in self-management in Tower Hamlets

Elizabeth Bayliss

Social Action for Health (SAfH) is a community development charity, with a focus on health inequalities, operating mainly in East London where there is the highest level of diversity in the country and the greatest wealth differential. High levels of poverty and high levels of unemployment are linked with high levels of chronic ill health, as established by the Joseph Rowntree Foundation (6) through their research series on the relationship between health and poverty. SAfH recognized that there is a relationship between the higher rates of general practitioner (GP) consultation associated with greater social and economic deprivation (7) reflected in Tower Hamlets (8) and peoples' low-level sense of being in control of their own health and well-being. We therefore felt that it would be a good idea to teach people how to take more control of managing their own health.

Background

In the year 2000, with funding from Tower Hamlets Social Services for promoting independence, we invited tenders from groups interested in running self-management courses with marginalized communities. The Long-Term Medical Conditions Alliance (LMCA) stepped forward. They trained Bengali speaking tutors and we converted the self-management manual so that it was culturally sensitive and appropriate in an Islamic context. At the same time, we sought a research body ready to evaluate this work and found Dr. Chris Griffiths, from the Centre for Health Sciences at Queen Mary's, University of London. He has gone on to undertake several research trials on self-management (9).

Profile of activity

Around 450 local Bengali men and women took part in the first courses in 2001. Each course was run by two trained tutors (themselves with a chronic condition) in mother tongue and on a gender specific basis. Since then, over 3,000 local people have taken part in courses we have run. We have trained over 60 people as tutors who run courses in their own language: Bengali, Sylheti, Somali, Turkish, Gugarati, French, Hindi, and English. Most of our courses are generic, for local people with a mix of chronic conditions; some are topped and tailed for people with a specific condition, such as pain, or asthma. We have developed our own self-management derivative on diabetes prevention, currently being adapted for work with obese people. We worked closely with the EPP to ensure that all our tutors were properly trained and reviewed and we actively supported the Steps to Quality (Ss2Q) initiative, on the basis that it is important that quality standards are maintained consistently across the field of lay-led self-management. Over the past couple of years, we have been commissioning independent trainers to teach new tutors and assess existing tutors. Currently, we are running around 70 courses a year for different PCTs or as the delivery agent in research trials on self-management. We organize a new training course once a year and a steady-stream of participants come to train as tutors after participating on a course.

What we have learnt

Increasing self-determination

Our focus on health inequalities leads us to work with people from marginalized communities and as a community development agency we are interested in self-determination. This means that we want to find ways by which people can take more control of their situations and the course does just that in relation to health and well-being. It is a useful tool in promoting self-determination in individuals. We find that this has beneficial ramifications across communities. Family members of participants have told us how the course benefited the whole family when Mum attended a course. Women participants talk about learning to sometimes say 'no' to family requests and taking time for themselves. Sons talk about their mums being more assertive, that family members know where they stand, and that their diet is better. Participants pass this knowledge on very quickly as they learn to identify their own needs, set their own goals and to negotiate. We hear how participants use their training in consultations with their GP. Being able to express their needs clearly improves their relationship with their GP and in turn increases their satisfaction with the NHS.

The power of role modelling

The courses are run by local people, themselves with chronic conditions, from the same community as the participants and they take place in mother tongue. This means the role modelling impact is great. The courses are inherently interactive, with the issues emerging from participants within the prescribed structure. Participants share their experiences and, because of shared culture, gender, and age group, a high level of social bonding can take place, leading to participants remaining in touch after the course has finished.

Participants are part of a movement

The mood at post-course certificate giving events, where people from different participating communities come together, is usually one of celebration. As many as 200 people come to these yearly events, keen to talk about the positive impact self-management has had on their lives, waving their certificates in the air with glee. We have learnt the power of holding gatherings and reunions to bring people back together again, and to do so cross-culturally so that people see themselves in a big context – they see themselves as part of a movement, as truly they are.

Benefits for all communities

We have found that people from all the different targeted communities enjoy learning how to take more control of their health. We have not found that traditional Muslim people are any less interested in taking more control than other people – far from it – a large proportion of our self-management work has been with Muslim people, so we would disagree with the view that Muslim people are fatalistic and passively accepting of ill-health. This view does not accord with our experience over the past 8 years at all.

Recruits for engagement in the public arena

We have also found that the courses throw up people interested in engaging in the public arena; people are keen to speak up about their experiences and help articulate problems so that others do not have to go through what they did.

Thus, we reap not only potential tutors from the courses, but also community activists who go on to represent their communities on various committees such as the Maternity Services Liaison Committee or as a School Governor. Many have gone on to train as SAfH Health Guides or Good Move! exercise tutors (10).

A call for social science research

Our purpose-designed database for our SAfH theme called 'Doing Your Part' has thousands of past participants on it. Many of these people are so positive about the benefits of the course that they remain in touch with SAfH for years after. We are hoping to attract a social scientist to evaluate the long-term impact of self-management, not so far adequately researched.

We wonder whether the motivational aspect of self-management can have a positive effect in the long-term on reducing the course of secondary conditions that result from poor management of a chronic condition. We have the contacts ready and waiting!

The database has revealed an interesting trend. If people are referred by their GP on to the course, they are less likely to complete than if self-referred or referred by a friend or relative. This indicates to us that there are further research questions here to be answered: do people referred by their GPs come on to the course because they are following orders? Do people who self-refer complete more frequently because they are more self-motivated? Does this difference suggest that the way self-management is promoted is important?

Practical lessons in working with diverse communities

We have learnt over the past 8 years how to recruit participants, on a culturally specific basis, through active outreach that involves training local people from the targeted communities who work in mother tongue. They go to the local people in their settings, working with and through existing community groupings, tapping into social networks, working with local radio to promote self-management involving Q&A and working with mosques and churches to reach people not connected to community groups.

We have also learnt to make direct contact early with anyone who is referred by a clinician to tell them about self-management. We build up a telephone relationship with people, keeping in touch sometimes for months before they can get onto a course that suits them. Leaflets are used to remind people of a personal contact they have had. They are never used as a primary means of communication.

In running courses, we have leant that the inspirational value of lay-led tutors cannot be overestimated. We pay tutors on a sessional basis that has meant that they are reliable and now very experienced. We support them, require them to refresh their skills and seek their views so that the work can be always improved.

Still questions after 15 years of experience

Phil Baker

Whatever the text book definition, the way self-management is seen and understood by different organizations is a significant determinant of how it is provided. Original attempts at definition have mostly come from the provider side not from the participants, who experience it in a much wider variety of ways. Listening to participants, and potential participants understanding and appreciation of the way it is seen and done provides the first key learning for provider organizations big and small.

Self-management is clearly related, but different from the broader 'self care' – it is how people manage and make the most of what they have and what may be limited by their condition(s). There is an implicit element of resisting the condition – not just being passive in the face of it's impacts and, crucially, in the face of what others say your expectations should be. Self-management is about how people pursue and try to meet their full range of bio-psycho-social needs; how they apply a whole range of coping strategies, external stimuli, and distractions to the focused management of the condition and its impacts. It is also how they best manage any sense of loss and/or being 'different' – so important for children and young people. For some, it includes aspects of anger management.

Self-management of a condition is influenced by many factors including:

♦ Length of time since diagnosis and embedded behaviours

♦ Access to information and medical support/advice

♦ Severity of the disease and co-morbidities

♦ Age, social support and level of education

Not all people want to, or can, self-manage their long term conditions (LTC). An individual's involvement in self-management is likely to fluctuate over time – it may increase, but it may also decrease. Young people, for most of whom 'not standing out' matters a lot, may be more influenced by a peer group than their condition; but support from parents and health professionals influences young people's compliance with ongoing self-management.

What matters is that people do not have to be alone in the task – the additional information, advice, training, and support from other people is crucial. Any successful approach to providing support and training for self-management has, therefore, to acknowledge and understand this complex set of practical and emotional elements for each individual. It also has to be set in the wider context of familial and social relationships and influences. In some cases, participants may experience very different cultural reactions to their conditions and the people who acquire them. It is evident from this that a training course, or it's equivalent, can only go so far in providing 'solutions' to the person in the middle of this complexity, and that a narrow range of training organizations is unlikely to present the broad range of understanding and provision required. Moreover, people should not just be provided with a course and then never seen or contacted again.

The course is probably best seen as a complimentary therapy. Complimentary, that is, to what the person already does and to the full range of formal health interventions, treatments and therapies. It is not in competition with, or has some claim to priority over these. Themes of complementarity and accompaniment (of the personal progress with the condition and through other support systems and treatment regimes) have emerged strongly from the experience of working with people with LTCs improve their self-management skills.

A snapshot from a range of participants at Arthritis Care courses shows a striking shift in language before and after attendance. In response to the question, *What does self-management mean to you?*

Dominant terminology	
Before the course:	After the course:
Coping	Managing
Being able to cope	Taking control

Over time, responses about motivation for attending and immediate impacts are remarkably consistent.
The top five reasons for attending a course?

1. Information

2. Prevent deterioration

3. Increase mobility

4. Cope with pain

5. Deal with depression

Top five most significant changes you have seen in yourself?

1. Increased self-confidence

2. Improved mobility

3. Positive attitude

4. No longer feel alone

5. Coping with pain

The notion of being 'trained' to self-manage is not that comfortable for some people; being 'educated' possibly even less so. The language and descriptors do bear on people's willingness to consider and participate in the courses on offer.

Delivering courses

The delivery of generic courses by disease-specific support organizations may be a factor in some people not identifying this as 'for them', if their condition is not the same. A small number of commissioners have raised this concern directly and it needs further examination – as do other potential barriers to participation such as, transport, jargon, and language. Some people are more attracted if the programme is co-branded with a local health agency or if held in health service premises. Others are actively discouraged by either or both of these.

It appears that self-management appeals to certain personality types. There may be clear predispositions that can be researched and better understood as to who are likely to be the best self-managers – the quiet stoics, the angry fighters, the fatalists, etc. What are the motivations/motivators that work best and how should potential beneficiaries be encouraged? Some of their disincentives are likely to be deeply rooted in gender, culture, and social background. Received wisdom, borne out in some measure by the make up of many courses, is that white, middle class women see themselves as good self-managers and so are attracted to the concept and the courses. If the participation in self-management courses is partly determined in that way, it raises a number of questions about how and when we start the process of attracting others who do not see themselves in that way, but who could potentially benefit most. Receiving and adjusting to a diagnosis is a process. People's ability to self–manage develops as part of a process. For many who either sign-up and then drop out, or who never sign-up at all, some form of informal introductory session may well help to explain and clarify purpose and content on the one side, and personal expectations on the other. Attempts to introduce these as part of funded or contracted provision have so far drawn a blank.

The context in which self-management training is offered can have a big impact on take-up. For example, government funded 'Back to Work' programmes for people with LTCs are intrinsically a good thing. However, for many, the whiff of coercion and withdrawal of benefits is not conducive to meaningful participation and many who could benefit do not. Independently funded courses offered to this group by Arthritis Care suffered from very low levels of participation for this express reason.

Where does self-management sit in the context of 'rights' under the NHS Constitution? Why shouldn't a person with an LTC demand their 'right' to good information and training on self-managing? There should be a clear entitlement to appropriately tailored services in the context of, and fully supported by, the 'community' around them. Optimizing the efficacy of self-management calls for a system-wide focus and approach.

What seems to work best?

1. Easy access to the right information, written from a user perspective, at the right time.
2. Where there is trust and empathy – being able to talk to others who understand a similar life with an LTC.
3. The right amount of time for the person: 6 weeks can be too long for some (fluctuating conditions) but shorter interventions do not necessarily allow the group dynamic and trust to develop fully.
4. Being 'trained' and supported by someone with a similar/same condition.
5. Ongoing advice and support from healthcare professionals and peers 'for the bad days' when the condition flares up or deteriorates.
6. Where there is understanding and allowances made – family, employers, fellow employees, educators, etc.

Awareness of the condition and its impacts among family, friends, etc. along with advice about fully supporting the individuals' efforts are essential components of the best and most successful self-management packages.

In many approaches to providing self-management training and support, there is a focus on how 'patients' need to change rather than how services need to develop in line with people's needs and expectations. There are a number of ways in which health agencies, working in partnership with local authorities and the voluntary sector, can best support people to self-manage their LTCs.

People rely on doctors for information about their health, in particular at diagnosis, so doctors themselves need to be properly informed about self-management education in order to support their patients.

In post-course questionnaires participants were asked: *Should this course be routinely prescribed by the GP?*

	Disease specific	Generic	Pain management
Yes	98%	90%	97%

Key themes for health service providers

- Develop incentives for health professionals to undertake learning.
- Skills development for the provision of support to self-management.
- Utilize nursing skills in patient education and self care by developing the role of nurses in managing chronic disease in, and across, practices.
- Focusing too narrowly on clinical outcomes misses the point.

   Change is needed in perception of broader value of self-management and the role of everyone involved.

- Commissioners should encourage far more self-management programmes as part of a wider strategy for LTCs. Costs involved for commissioners should be seen as a good investment to gain a long-term benefit.

National guidance is needed on the balance of disease specific and generic provision. There does not appear to be conclusive proof that any disease specific course is best for everybody. Arthritis Care has experience of both responses; some people with arthritis preferring the mixture of experiences among participants on generic courses, while others would only consider a course if it was arthritis specific. Such research that has been done demonstrates rough parity in outcomes for both (for the aspects that were researched at least).

Good self-management training costs – be that recruiting and training tutors, whether staff or volunteers, assessing and maintaining their accreditation, planning and delivering, or monitoring and reporting. In reality, few organizations will be making any money from it – the prices (tariffs) being offered by commissioners do not meet the costs for many providers, so de facto subsidies are in place. In theory, this gives advantage to smaller community-based providers, but there's a quality threshold to be maintained and formal, paid for third party accreditation/certification is coming.

Is providing self-management a priority for all patient organizations?

Many would say not, with scarce resources focused on lobbying for improved health provision. For many, it is a bit of a distraction with potential to only reach a few compared to benefits for the majority if lobbying is successful. But participation by people with LTCs often begins a process of engagement that can lead to peer support groups and acting as 'Expert Users' in the wider process of service change and improvement. The transformational experience that many people undergo can generate a powerful impulse to become more involved and to 'give something back'.

If there is a true 'patient pathway' that begins with diagnosis and continues to end of life care, then many organizations like Arthritis Care should see their role and services as entirely complimentary and meriting full integration and acknowledgement for their value. That said, we should be careful not to over claim for it. Not everyone derives equal benefit and the sense of continuity that the best care packages predict is not always possible with the relatively scarce resources at the disposal of many providers. Scaling up this time consuming and expensive service is a major challenge. Government aspirations around increased use of self-management, often for rather narrowly focused financial reasons, will never be fully realized if there isn't a purposeful move to 'whole person/whole system' thinking that drives long term, properly funded programmes. In the absence of any further central government interventions driving this, it is left to the other actors to forge the approach. The barriers are not insurmountable but each one needs to let go of certain things and find common ground – providers should look beyond narrow concerns about competition; commissioners should look beyond fulfilling mere numerical targets; health professionals need to look beyond the surgery/consulting room and see real value in what can be done elsewhere, with different but complimentary approaches.

The online opportunity

Ian McNeil

On a T-Trainer Course training at Stanford (2002), I observed what Stanford was doing with their online version of the course. I thought then that it had the potential to fit in with modern life styles and had especial potential for remote and rural areas. In devising the project, we wanted to recreate the experience of attending a local course. Each online course has two 'moderators' (the equivalent of community tutors) or, in EPP terminology, 'facilitators'. I moderated several courses for Stanford in 2003/2004 and became the Project Manager for EPP online in 2004. The established Stanford approach included a friendly attitude to enquirers; a system of checks and safeguards that maintained a safe and supportive online environment; and a greater opportunity for mutual support than I'd previously experienced. We all wondered if British reserve might make the English trial less successful than that in the US.

Before arriving as Project Manager, Katy Plant and the team at PERC had made many adjustments to the US course to accommodate linguistic, cultural, and legal differences. Eventually, after much work with colleagues in the EPP and Ayesha Dost at the DoH, we obtained ethics approval in the USA and the UK. We leant heavily on established good practice for working with volunteers and on experience of working with self-management tutors in the UK voluntary sector. We attempted to comply with the principles of the quality assurance framework for EPP known as SS2Q (Stepping Stones to Quality).

Working with the NHS Prescription Pricing Authority, we developed a detailed recruitment package for aspiring online facilitators ensuring fair and impartial selection. Trained facilitators operated in pairs on each course much as course tutors do for community courses. As their manager I was acting as a 'SuperUser' daily moderating their work to ensure protocols were observed so that courses were run uniformly for the benefit and safety of participants. A system of pairing experienced with new facilitators was introduced to cope with the expanding workload. As facilitators became more adept fewer referrals were made to the Project Manager. In later stages, an accomplished facilitator, cleared by Stanford Ethics Board, was able to deputise for me. We learned that the role of 'SuperUser' needs to be shared to avoid the stress of providing 24/7 availability. Throughout each course, telephone conferences for facilitators were held to reinforce good practice.

This project was sufficiently financed to allow full discussion of the processes and learning we were experiencing. Difficulties with the website were dealt with expeditiously by Stanford as were suggestions from facilitators. As experience grew, protocols were developed for identifying any 'inflammatory' posts to the Discussion Centre and for addressing concern for participants who might be at risk of possible suicide or self-harm. This very detailed and specific protocol, developed with senior colleagues in the UK and at Stanford, was welcomed by the facilitators. Some expressed a need for similar clarity for community tutors.

We deliberately developed a sense of community among the widely scattered facilitators by bringing them together on three occasions to promote good practice and develop teamwork. At the final event, a celebration, where the facilitators expressed their satisfaction, most wished to remain involved. Crucially, we learned that a comprehensive framework of support for the facilitators was fundamental to achieving high levels of involvement by online participants.

Having spaces for only 600 people, we opted for a relatively low-key approach to participant recruitment to avoid creating a demand for the online course that the planned pilot could not satisfy. Leaflets and posters were produced for use by the EPP staff and both Ethics Boards approved these materials. The principle publicity mechanism was the EPP itself but in addition, a Reference Group of key stakeholders including voluntary sector partners was established. The new EPP online facilitators proved to be enthusiastic advocates and took every opportunity to disseminate information about the project. We also contacted other frequently used online health sites.

Features for online courses

From observations and experience of the 27 courses in the EPP Online Pilot, I believe that a number of possibilities deserve further investigation.

Participants are willing to use the (online) Discussion and Suggestion Boards to disclose much more about themselves than occurred on community courses, and do so much earlier. This was unexpected and dispelled any initial concerns we had about 'natural British Reserve'. From my own experience, there was a more vigorous participation by participants than I had experienced when moderating online courses in USA.

- They have the potential to reach a much younger section of the population than community courses. We attracted a younger age profile than expected and many were students or working.

- They might represent an attractive proposition to employers needing to retain experienced staff who have LTCs. Individuals who had learnt self-management skills earlier in life might stay in employment longer.

- They could be an additional point of access to self-management and provide means to enable those currently on benefits to prepare for return to work.

- Its flexibility allowed for people accessing the course whilst on holiday in Europe and the USA.

- They provide an ideal means for refresher courses that could be valuable for people experiencing a 'down cycle' in their LTC.

- There's an opportunity to establish an online self-management community where 'graduates' could 'meet' for mutual support and encouragement. A start could be made on 'linking the thinking' helping to pull together diverse strands of activity and helping people to make sense of the plethora of information and resources available.

- If we can generate such interest with a sustained but low-key approach, there can be little doubt that we could generate significantly greater demand with a few more resources and higher profile 'campaign'.

Three concluding observations

There is no wealth but life.

John Ruskin (1819–1900)

There are opportunities as well as dangers in the emerging quality and support framework for lay-led self-management. While the development of standards appears to be intrinsically 'a good thing', any standard must be seen to be an 'enabler' that increases provision and accessibility of self-management, reduces current inequities, and more than just another costly 'hoop to jump through' that reduces that availability. Standards need to be flexible enough to recognize the different ways of achieving the same goal yet accommodating emerging and developing practice in different parts of the country. They must be seen to have relevance amid the seemingly endless plethora of standard setting and avoid yet another contribution to over regulation. Finally, they must not contribute to a perception of professionalization of delivery that would lead to the very real danger of losing the passion and enthusiasm that is such a valuable hallmark of self-management in the UK.

> Life is about more than just maintaining oneself, it is about extending oneself. Otherwise living is only not dying.
>
> Simone de Beauvoir (1908–1986)

I have heard so much about 'limitations' of the online course: these might be due to deficiencies of IT skill or access to it, or its unsuitability for older people. I can emphatically reject all of these as limitations. Contact with organizations like Age Concern explodes the myth. Access to IT continues to improve – it is available in libraries, Internet Cafes, community, and even village halls. Moreover, there are many imaginative solutions to address lack of access. Given the growing importance of Corporate Social Responsibility (CSR) to organizations and its inclusion in an increasing number of annual reports, the options to share IT should be explored. Low cost eco-friendly solutions are there – we just need to implement them.

> A vision without a task is but a dream, a task without a vision is drudgery, a vision and a task is the hope of the world.
>
> From a church in Sussex ca.1730

Finally, my experience of the online pilot was a perfect reflection of this quote. We all had shared a vision about extending access to self-management and willingly accepted the task of making that vision a reality. I believe, as do those involved in delivering the project, that we were successful and the research published in 2008 confirms that view(12). I hope that the online course finds its rightful place as an important means of delivering self-management to people throughout the UK, complementing existing provision and offering wider access to self-management.

Maintaining standards

Jane Cooper

Stepping Stones to Quality (Ss2Q) is the first and currently, the only quality assurance system for providers of Stanford's self-management courses.

The seeds of Ss2Q were sown within Arthritis Care in the early 1990s when they developed a basic framework for training and supporting volunteers delivering the Challenging Arthritis course. In the late 1990s, the Long-term Medical Conditions Alliance (LMCA – now National Voices) was awarded funds by the Department of Health to explore the use of self-management among its member organizations. In the Long-term Illness (Lill) project, the Chronic Disease Self-Management Course (CDSMC) was delivered to a heterogeneous group of people living with LTCs from the LMCA member organizations. (The group included some people supporting individuals living with rarer conditions.)

LMCA recruited and supported eight of its member organizations (6) to establish their own self-management programmes using the CDSMC. Other partners included Arthritis Care, using their expertise to train and accredit tutors; the Charities Evaluation Services supporting the development of robust monitoring and evaluation processes; and the Psychosocial Research Centre at Coventry University (now the Applied Research Centre in Health and Life Sciences) that undertook research on the medium term affects of the course on participants.

LMCA requested that participating organizations nominate a Coordinator, responsible for the day-to-day management of the programme and participation in the facilitated CDSMC Network. This was essentially a forum for coordinators to seek practical support. The realities of supporting people living with LTCs to deliver scheduled courses (for example, they are sometimes ill at short notice) and finding enough participants, meant that they were very soon using the Network as a market place to exchange 'tricks of the trade' and negotiate reciprocal sharing of resources. Membership of the Network was dependent on adherence to the principle that local courses were only be delivered by people living with LTCs.

In 2001, the first attempt was made by Network members to record the good practice that had developed as common knowledge. The introduction of the NHS EPP in 2002 added impetus to this process, as it became apparent that the proposed scale and diversity of operations would be such that sharing of good practice would need to be carried out on a more systematic basis.

Over the next 3 years, the NHS EPP worked collaboratively with third sector organizations (TSOs) and PCTs to articulate the 'golden rules' for developing, implementing, and sustaining lay-led self-management programmes. A cross sector Quality Assurance Group (QAG)[1] was established to support and oversee this work.

In 2005, Stepping Stones to Success (9) was published. This document was endorsed by 18 organizations involved in supporting or delivering

Stanford programmes. Ss2Q contains guidelines on developing and implementing programmes with the aim of ensuring that all local lay-led courses are delivered to a consistently high standard across the country. The Network identified four steps to developing high-quality lay-led self-management programmes:

Step 1	Adhere to the core values and principles of lay-led self-management
Step 2	Generate support for your programme within your organization and communities you serve
Step 3	Identify a self-management coordinator
Step 4	Recruit, train and support people living with LTCs, and those who care for them, to deliver lay-led self-management programmes

Stepping Stones to Success has a companion portfolio of web-based supporting documentation containing all the templates developed by members of the CDSMC Network to facilitate the recruitment, training, and support of tutors to deliver community courses (10).

During 2006, a sub-group of QAG was established to work with The Health Care Standards Unit and an independent evaluation agency, to broaden the content of Stepping Stones to Success into a quality framework. The result was Stepping Stones to Quality (Ss2Q) (11). Ss2Q is a straightforward and practical self-assessed quality assurance framework. Its purpose is to ensure that all lay-led self-management programmes covered by Stanford licences are implemented consistently and effectively to the benefit of people living with LTCs. Ss2Q builds upon the four Stepping Stones to Success. Within each of the four steps, there are four sections that relate to different aspects of managing and delivering a lay-led self-management programme:

Programme management – What is being done?

Programme design – How will it be done?

Programme delivery – Who is going to do it?

Programme evaluation – Did it make a difference?

The result is 16 standards that focus on the things organizations need to do in order to run programmes well and achieve good results for participants. There is a series of questions organizations can use to self-assess and they are encouraged to maintain a portfolio of evidence to demonstrate that they are meeting the standards.

While there is widespread support for Ss2Q among the provider community in England, there is less certainty as to the extent to which people living with LTCs are driving the development and implementation of self-management programmes within organizations. It is anticipated that this issue will be addressed by the introduction of the Ss2Q Quality Mark accreditation scheme for provider agencies. This will provide tangible evidence of involvement of people living with LTCs in the strategic and operational mechanics of programmes. The creation of the Ss2Q Quality Mark will be taken forward by a new independent Quality Institute for Self-Management Education and Training (QISMET). A consortium of Arthritis Care, Diabetes UK, Expert Patients Programme Community Interest Company (EPP–CIC), Macmillan Cancer Support, volunteer tutors and PCTs, laid the foundations and developed a business plan in consultation with stake holders, which led to the award of a 3-year grant from the Department of Health Third Sector Investment Programme in March 2009. It is to establish a values driven membership organization that will be responsible for:

◆ Developing and managing standards and accreditation processes for a range of self-management education and training services

◆ Supporting self-management education and training providers to build capacity and expertise for continuous improvement

◆ Providing membership-based information and supports services

◆ Promoting the involvement of people living with LTCs, professionals, and organizations in the development and implementation of self-management education and training

The development of Ss2Q and greater use of self-management for people living with LTCs has coincided with, and been driven by, a national policy context in which self-management and self care are at the heart of meeting the future health care needs of an ageing population living with more LTCs. Initiatives such as patient and public involvement, self care, choice, care closer to home, world class commissioning, and the identification of continuous improvement of quality of care as the guiding principle of the NHS all provide the ongoing rationale for the further development of standards and accreditation for self-management education and training provision. Ss2Q has set the benchmark for the development of standards in self-management. QISMET will aspire to continue in the spirit of partnership epitomized by the development of Ss2Q, supporting an increase in the provision high-quality self-management services led by and for people living with LTCs.

Endnotes

1 QAG included representatives from NHS EPP, voluntary sector organisations, Primary Care Trusts, volunteer tutors and the Lay Led Self-Management Network (the successor to the CDSMC Network).

References

1. Our Health, Our Care, Our Say: *a new direction for community services.* 2006, White Paper, TSO (The Stationery Office) London.

2. Kennedy A., Reeves D., Bower P., Lee V., Middleton E., Richardson G., et al. (2007a). The effectiveness and cost effectiveness of a national lay led self care support programme for patients with long-term conditions: a pragmatic randomised controlled trial. *J Epidemiol Community Health.* **61**: 254–61.

3. High quality care for all: NHS Next Stage Review final report, 2008, Command paper, Professor the Lord Darzi of Denham KBE , TSO (The Stationery Office), London.

4. Cooper J., Thompson J. (2005) Stepping Stones to Success: An implementation framework for lay led self-management programmes. Department of Health.

5. Expert Patients Programme Community Interest Company. Stepping Stones Supporting Information. Available at www.expertpatients.co.uk.

6. Expert Patients Programme Community Interest Company (2007) Stepping Stones to Quality a quality framework and audit tool for lay led self-management programmes. EPP–CIC.

7. Salway S., Platt L., Chowbey P., Harris K., Bayliss E. (2007) *Long-Term Ill Health, Poverty and Ethnicity.* York: Joseph Rowntree Foundation.

8. Goddard M., Smith P. (1998) *Equity of Access to Health Care.* York: University of York.

9. East London and the City Strategic Health Authority (1998) *Independent Inquiry into inequalities in Health Report, Part 2.* London: The National Health Service, ELCHA .

10. Griffiths CJ., Ramsay J., Motlib M., Azad A., Begum R., Garrett M., Barlow J., Feder G., Elderidge S. (2003) *Expert Bangladeshi patients? Interim Results for a Randomised Trial of Lay-Led Self Management in Bangladeshis with Chronic Disease. Or Can California Come to East London?* London: Centre for Health Sciences, University of London (QMUL).

11. Lis Retzmann (2009) *Good Move! Steps to a healthier life, SAfH report 1.* London: Social Action for Health.

12. Lorig KR., Ritter PL., Dost A., Plant K., Laurent DD., McNeil I. (2008) The expert patients programme online, a 1-year study of an Internet-based self-management programme for people with long-term conditions. *Chronic Illness.* **4**(4): 247–56. DOI:http://dx.doi.org/10.1177/1742395308098886

Chapter 7

The value of self-management: Retrieving a sense of self: the loss and reconstruction of a life

Patrick Hill and Mike Osborn

Since 2000, new health policy and service provision for people with long-term health conditions in England, including the NHS Expert Patients Programme (EPP), would appear to indicate a health and social care system taking positive steps towards providing a more empowering form of support for people with long-term health conditions (e.g. 1–3). However, despite a growing awareness of the need for people with long-term conditions to be empowered, to have more control over their health, policy makers and service providers have demonstrated little understanding of the complexity or timescale of the journey that enables people, with potentially debilitating long-term conditions, become effective self-managers.

Despite numerous evaluations and research trials providing evidence for the efficacy of various interventions (e.g. 4), the actual needs of people with long-term conditions were not clarified by the traditional (quantitative) research literature which focused on outcomes rather than the process of coping. Conrad's (5) commentary on qualitative research in chronic illness suggested that the major issues in managing long-term conditions are social, rather than medical, and thus qualitative research 'appears to be particularly well-suited for studying and understanding the subjective and processural (or changing) aspects of illness'. (p. 1257).

To this end, an increasing number of qualitative studies of people's experience of living with long-term conditions have been published in recent years, e.g. in pain (6, 7); vitiligo (8); chronic bronchitis (9); HIV (17); and coping with myocardial infarction (10), Barlow et al. (11) have explored people's experience of self-management.

The aim of the qualitative study reported here was to retrospectively explore the process of acquiring the skills of self-management and its impact on people's coping. The experiences of a sample of empowered participants who had achieved a recognized level of confidence in self-management of long-term health conditions provided the focus for the research. Their achievement was defined by their particular role, in that they were established as trainers or tutors in the NHS 'EPP' (1).

Participants

In the summer of 2004, after obtaining ethical approval, participants were recruited from the national group of EPP trainers and volunteer tutors. Participants were interviewed at a convenient time and place, which in most cases was their own home. The group of 6 participants consisted of 3 men and 3 women aged between 35 and 55 years, with a variety of long-term conditions including rheumatoid arthritis, back pain, multiple sclerosis, epilepsy, and endometriosis.

Data collection and analysis

Interpretative Phenomenological Analysis (IPA) was chosen as an appropriate methodology as it is: 'specifically designed to explore the meaningful experiences of individuals as they deal with aspects of their life, allowing them to describe how a disease or other life-event has affected them over time' (12, p. 215). The nature of this type of exploration of the person's experience can be described as phenomenological, that is, it is concerned with the individual's particular account of their reality (Smith 1995). However, IPA is also interpretative in that the analysis allows for the researcher's interpretation of the narratives.

The participants were invited to take part in a single semi-structured interview, proposed as the exemplary method of data collection for studies using IPA by Smith and Osborn (13). Consideration was given to the recommended strategies to ensure credibility and coherence in the data collection and analysis (14, 15).

A schedule was used as a prompt to guide the interview to areas the researcher felt were important. Participants were encouraged to tell the story of their personal experiences of living with their condition(s) and developing the skills of self-management.

The interviews were audio-recorded and notes were taken. At the end of the interview, participants were asked to reflect on the interview process. After the recorded interviews were transcribed verbatim by a typist, the individual transcripts were sent to the participants who were asked to comment and respond to some further reflective questions, following the suggestions made in the guidelines for qualitative research proposed by Elliot et al. (14) and Reicher (15).

The transcripts were subjected to a qualitative thematic analysis to categorize and explore the data for common themes and patterns so as to produce a coding frame. The coding frame and two of the transcripts were given to the second author, experienced both in qualitative analysis using IPA and in self-management of long-term conditions. He verified the grounding of the thematic analysis in the raw data and made suggestions about the thematic structure.

The analysis was effectively a two-stage process, which comprised identification of themes followed by a more detailed interpretative or conceptual analysis, as described by Nicolson and Anderson (9). IPA provided the basis for the conceptual analysis.

The analysis presented here has been written up around one core theme, '*Retrieving a sense of self: the loss and reconstruction of a life*'. The participants described a process of change in their sense of self over-time (independent of the progress of their illness) whereby important aspects of their sense of self and identity were lost and then retrieved to some degree, through the experience of self-managing their condition and support they received, including acting as participants and deliverers of the EPP. The retrieved or reconstructed self was not identical to the pre-illness self, but it was familiar in some way, acknowledged the long-term nature of their illness and involved some notion of agency and social value.

Retrieving a sense of self: the loss and reconstruction of a life

Integral to each of the participants' experience of their condition and later success with self-management was, first, an inexorable and powerless sense of the gradual disassembling of their sense of self, as part of a descent into a disabled and distressed state and loss of their former lives, followed by a period of recovery and the emergence of a more positive contemporary social self or a new 'life', that was both familiar and yet different than before.

The participants felt they had little discretion over the early stages of the process and described themselves as if they were observing from a helpless position. Despite their best attempts to resist the initial decline, they gradually lost the ability to fulfil their former social roles, or make sense of or regulate their behaviour or emotions. They described themselves as being quietly overwhelmed by their illness. This period of their lives was described as, 'the lowest of times', it varied in length and quality, but each participant described a similar period of decline into a powerless and paralyzing sense of despair. Eventually, facilitated by self-management, this process began to reverse and was followed by a period of recovery that they described as 'getting my life back'.

The loss of self – 'the lowest of times'

Charlie, having begun the interview quite tentatively, became more enthusiastic in his focus on this process of decline and described the inexorable deterioration of his sense of self quite explicitly, emphasizing his powerlessness and the level of despair involved:

> just going down and down and down yeah.... I could see that getting worse and worse ... there didn't seem to be any way of getting out of it ... its sometimes difficult looking back on that sort of time and thinking how did I feel? Difficult to remember what it's like but also it was a hard time to sort of be in
>
> Charlie

In his use of repetition at the beginning of the excerpt, Charlie added extra emphasis to his statement. In phrases such as '*down and down and down*' and '*getting worse and worse*' he conveyed, in very simple terms, the powerlessness he felt as his sense of self deteriorated. The process Charlie described took place over a lengthy period of 4–6 years and the return phase was defined as getting back to a notion of '*normality*'. Normality wasn't defined by any normative criteria, but by the return of a more familiar personal sense of self and lifestyle:

> It's about four years before I went there and two years like having to use self-management tools. I was a long way getting down to where I was and you know it's a long way back up to get back to a sort of semblance of normality ... the old me
>
> Charlie

For '*normality*', Charlie referred to a return to a more familiar experience of himself, '*the old me*'. The contemporary normality involved experiences of the self that were recognizable to some degree, but now also involved having a long-term condition. This suggested a change in his resistance to accepting the permanence of his condition. This resistance was shared by many of the participants:

> I'd have found that really interesting, not when I was going through the dark days but as I was crawling out of them, to have gone to a pain clinic where there'd be that sort of information and talks available about illness behaviours and noises you make when you move and all that sort of stuff ... but if they'd tried to do that when I was really ill I would have hit them ... timing's everything !
>
> Susan

Susan, like Charlie, described how making progress was very difficult and something that only proceeded slowly. She described how she '*crawled*' along and how in the early stages this was a reluctant and resistant process. She felt quite strongly that, had she been offered self-management too early, she would have seen it as an unacceptable and coercive force and resisted it aggressively, '*lashed out*'. In rejecting the chronicity of her condition, she also rejected any offers of help.

Being approached with the right therapeutic message at the right time was important to her and being given the wrong message too early would have been problematic and far from benign, compounding her loss of self and leaving her in a more disabled, alienated, and distressed state.

Turning a corner

Each of the participants looked back and identified a point where their situation had changed for the better. Gerald described his experience of learning to live with and manage his condition as a '*return journey*', a recovery from a period of decline and disintegration:

> One of things I noticed on this journey … that is of no significance at all, except that it was very important, I started wearing aftershave again. There was a time when I was so despondent…. If a pair of trousers was comfortable, if a pair of shoes was comfortable then that was all that mattered and the colour of the trousers and the shoes didn't matter and you certainly weren't going to wear aftershave … now there comes a point on your return journey when you do begin caring about those things, not as much as before, they still have to be comfortable, but you worry and you start wearing aftershave again and … you begin to … the rich tapestry of life rather than just anything will keep me warm!
>
> Gerald

For Gerald, this process was evidenced in his approach to self care and grooming. He described a descent into self-neglect, where very little mattered regarding his appearance, followed by a return to some form of self care and self-interest. More specifically, this involved the re-emergence of a pride in his appearance and an interest and concern in how he presented himself to the outside world. In anticipation of re-engaging with more of his social world, becoming less withdrawn, he began to care about what others might think of him.

His mood was, in his words, 'despondent' and the related self neglect prompted a utilitarian approach to his appearance, where practical comfort took priority and little else held any positive meaning. He had retreated from almost all social contact and simply dressed to satisfy the physical demands of his environment. As he began to make progress, the social meaning of his appearance re-emerged in the form of a '*worry*', or a concern about how he might appear to others. As his self neglect receded, he began to groom himself again and returned to some of his familiar practices. For Gerald, this involved wearing aftershave, which to him was the apogee of his journey, the point at which he felt he had secured a palpable sense of change and progress. He began to consider his appearance, care for himself and, it could be argued, see himself in a more positive light. He doesn't describe applying aftershave in a defensive way, as a mask to hide behind, but as something that denoted his re-emergence into a social world and return from a period of self-neglect.

Gerald was clear in his account that he felt his return journey did not involve an immaculate restoration of his previous life or self, '*it's not the old me*', but that instead it represented a return to a more familiar state. A more recognizable state where he experienced a richer or more meaningful life, one that he described as '*a rich tapestry*', rather that a utilitarian, monochromatic, or one-dimensional life, where only '*warmth*' mattered and only basic physical needs were satisfied.

Charlie, like Gerald, recalled a similar point which he felt represented a change in his situation and an indication that he had improved:

> It's like a tool a stepping tool for me really to get back into full time work ... from being near enough housebound ... you know there's certain things I forget – I went to a barbers and got me hair cut the other day. First time in five years I've ever sat in a barbers

Charlie

Like Gerald, Charlie's account of making progress involved moving from a socially withdrawn, 'housebound' state, dominated by illness, to being more focused on the possibility of achieving something in the future, in his case, getting '*back into full time employment*'. His progress was also marked by a return to an interest in his appearance and a visit to the barbers. Charlie went from a situation of overwhelming disability, unable to do anything more than tolerate his illness, to contemplating a re-entry into a social setting and a re-emergence of a pride in his appearance. Both Charlie and Gerald described their progress in relation to their social-presentation and social engagement and made little reference to any change in their condition or their disability. As their situation improved, their attention broadened from simply enduring their condition and satisfying their most basic and physical needs to considering their appearance and their place within their social world. They had moved from enduring a disabled state of surviving, where their consciousness was overwhelmed by feelings of powerlessness, hopelessness, and withdrawal, to having some kind of meaningful vision of a future that they could engage with. One which included a valued sense of self, a 'me' that they could take out and present to the social world and did not need to conceal. The person was beginning to re-emerge.

The reconstruction – 'getting their life back'

Each of the participants had experienced a sense of progress and recovery. The reconstruction was a lengthy and difficult process that included the physical, emotional, social, and psychological aspects of their condition working in combination:

> Well the surgery and medication have, you know, without a doubt had a major impact. You know without having the right surgeon and finding medication that seemed to work.... So it isn't just an emotional shift even though I believe that's a very big part of it as well, it does for me go hand in hand with the treatment I got medically.
>
> Susan

Susan acknowledged the reciprocal and dynamic relationship between each of the bio-psycho-social factors involved in her progress. The reconstruction of her sense of self was not an isolated, purely intra-psychic phenomenon and in the final stage of reconstruction she described the emergence of a new self, socially situated, of '*growing into something else*' and '*returning a bit to the world*'.

> It's a real cliché that people say that they got their life back or got a life and it does feel like that, but it also feels like a different life ... self-management gave me a way of you know growing into something else ... and you know returning a bit to the world ... it really feels like a before and after for me
>
> Susan

Susan took some pride in the reconstruction process and described how self-management helped her to achieve it and experience a more acceptable self, and a different life, '*feels like a before and after for me*'. The other participants were also empowered in this process, and one change the EPP helped them feel was that they could help themselves and were not powerless observers of their lives, '*I could do this myself, something I could do*'.

> It was like a feeling of empowerment as the weeks went on, I could actually do this myself, summat I could do, not having to rely on the doctors to help me you know - that hadn't worked for four years then.... So I had four years of not being helped and it sort of all seemed to be that I could do something myself.
>
> Charlie

The participants began to feel less passive and more proactive. In this way, the new emergent self was more purposeful, empowered, and socially valued:

> I 'spose perhaps I didn't think much before but its made me think ... well I've got to be proactive and do things myself - not wait for other people to you know ... do things ... and to take responsibility ... for it and you know and to decide what I thinks best for me and what suits me best.
>
> Mary

The participants all looked back and were struck by how they had changed over time, perhaps against their will. This was evident in their behaviour, their approach to their appearance and interpersonal relationships. For Susan, this was evident in a more assertive and secure approach to her consultations with health professionals:

> Thinking that bloody well wasn't ok and going and talking to my doctor about it. I really wasn't happy with this consultation – this is how I saw it and this is what was said ... but I thought, God I wouldn't of ever gone back to the doctor in the old days I would have just cried more in the car park so I felt like I'd really changed in thinking they were always right

Susan

As Susan's situation improved, she became more active in her own care and confident in the value of her own opinion compared to others. She now felt less inadequate and inferior in the face of health professionals. Her earlier experiences were anti-therapeutic and had left her feeling more distressed and hopeless, crying in her car. She now had the confidence to consider her own opinion as legitimate and to challenge the views of others. In this way, like Charlie and Gerald, she emerged from a more withdrawn and insecure position to engage with a more social world.

The participants described how they had felt propelled through a similar process of change, a 'return journey'. In each case, they made no reference to any change or spontaneous improvement in their medical condition, but a change in their disability and distress and more explicitly how they viewed themselves in a physical and psychosocial context. As the interviews progressed, they articulated this process in more detail and the notion of a return journey was described further as a process of first losing, then retrieving, a sense of self and identity. The new self was familiar, but not identical to their pre-condition self and enabled them to live with their condition more therapeutically and function better in a social context.

Feedback from participants

The participants' feedback was consistently positive about receiving the transcripts of their interviews. The responses also reinforced the importance of the theme 'Being on a journey'.

> It was good to see the transcript as the interview with you enabled me to reflect around where I was – how far I have come – where I am today and to some extent where I want to go in the future.

Robert

Conclusions

The participants in this study reported finding value, meaning, fulfilment, and empowerment through the development of self-management and their role in the EPP. Their reflections on their journey indicated that they were aware of the changes they had experienced and that they had emerged from this process as different people.

A subtle and elusive process has been described. That is, the process interpreted as core changes to the self that occur during a metamorphic journey from wellness to illness, to self-management and coping, re-emerging as a new person, the same but different and in control of their new lives.

The learning from this is that health and social care services would appear to need to widen their vision of the support needed by people with long-term conditions. What has been clarified is the need to move beyond simply addressing identified physical, emotional, psychological, and social needs, through single short-term interventions. Interventions need to support a process of empowerment, enabling people to make a choice about taking control, through appreciating the value of their own ability to self-manage, 'rebuild' their sense of self and establish new and valid roles in society.

The suggestion is that a flexible range of provision is required to support people through their journey. It seems unlikely that health professionals alone will be able to offer the support that will empower many people as many of the important determinants of effective self-management, such as employment and social support lie outside of health care.

For self-management support to be an empowering process, it needs to be understood by health and social care services, not as an education that transforms people with long-term conditions into 'better' people, but as one that enables people to retrieve their sense of self through a long process that is enabling, liberating, energizing, and supportive.

Acknowledgements

Dr. Ian Bennun for support, advice, and several rewrites. The interview participants for giving their time and their personal stories, and in doing so opening the shutters and letting in the light.

References

1. Department of Health (2001) *The Expert Patient: A New Approach to Chronic Disease Management for the 21st Century.* London: Department of Health.
2. Department of Health (2005) *Self Care - A Real Choice Self Care Support - A Practical Option.* London: Department of Health.

3. Department of Health (2006) *Our Health, Our Care, Our Say: A New Direction for Community Services.* London: Department of Health.

4. Morley S., Ecclestone C., Williams AC de C. (1999) Systematic review of randomised controlled trials of cognitive behaviour therapy and behaviour therapy for chronic pain in adults excluding headache. *Pain.* **80:** 1–13.

5. Conrad P. (1990) Qualitative research on chronic illness: A commentary on method and conceptual development. *Social Science and Medicine.* **30:** 1257–63.

6. Aldrich S., Eccleston C. (2000) Making sense of everyday pain. *Social Science Medicine.* **50**(11): 1631–41.

7. Osborn M., Smith JA. (1998) The personal experience of chronic benign lower back pain: an interpretative phenomenological analysis. *British Journal of Health Psychology.* **3:** 65–83.

8. Thompson AR., Kent G. (2001) Adjusting to disfigurement: Processes involved in dealing with being visibly different. *Clinical Psychology Review.* **21:** 663–82.

9. Nicolson P., Anderson P. (2003) Quality of Life, distress and self-esteem: A focus group study of people with chronic bronchitis. *British Journal of Health Psychology.* **8**(3): 251–70.

10. Hogg NM., Garratt V., Shaw SK., Tagney J. (2007) It has certainly been good to talk: An interpretative phenomenological analysis of coping with myocardial infarction. *British Journal of health Psychology.* **12:** 651–62.

11. Barlow JH., Bancroft GV., Turner AP. (2004) Volunteer, lay tutors' experiences of the Chronic Disease Self-Management Course: being valued and adding value. *Health Education Research Advance Access* 2005 April; **20**(2): 128–36.

12. Thompson AR., Kent G., Smith JA. (2002) Living with Vitiligo: Dealing with Difference. *British Journal of Health Psychology.* **7**(2): 213–25.

13. Smith, JA. (1995) Semi-structured interviewing and qualitative analysis. In JA. Smith, R. Harre & V. Langerhove (Eds.), *Rethinking methods in psychology* (pp. 9-26). London: Sage.

14. Smith JA., Osborn M. (2003) Interpretative Phenomenological Analysis. In: Smith J (editor) *Qualitative Psychology a Practical Guide to Research Methods,* 51–80. London: Sage.

15. Elliot R., Fischer CT., Rennie DL. (1999) Evolving guidelines for publication of qualitative research studies in psychology and related fields. *British Journal of Clinical Psychology.* **38**(3): 215–30.

16. Reicher S. (2000) Against methodolatry: Some comments on Elliott, Fischer and Rennie. *British Journal of Clinical Psychology.* **39:** 1–6.

17. Flowers P., Duncan B., Knussen C. (2003) Re-appraising HIV testing: An exploration of the psychosocial costs and benefits associated with learning one's HIV status in a purposive sample of Scottish gay men. *British Journal of Health Psychology.* **8:** 179–94.

Chapter 8

Self-management and government policy

David Colin-Thomé OBE

Efforts are underway in the UK as elsewhere to improve the management of long-term conditions with an emphasis on enhancing patients' confidence and skills for self-management and involvement in decision-making. This chapter will briefly describe the current government policy designed to improve health outcomes for those members of the public who live with a long-term condition. It will also equally briefly describe the current and potential role of general medical practice in addressing the care needs of these patients.

Prioritizing care for those who have a long-term condition was announced by the English Department of Health in The NHS Improvement Plan published in 2004 (1), although elements of the policy set out there predated the Plan. These elements include the Expert Patient Programme (2), inspired by the chronic disease self-management programme developed by Kate Lorig at Stanford (3), and the new contract for general medical practitioners that provides financial incentives to GPs and their teams to improve the quality of chronic care (4). The NHS Improvement Plan was significant in bringing together these and other initiatives.

Prioritizing was an explicit recognition of the changing burden of disease in the population arising from an ageing population. Data (5) indicates that over 30% of people report that they have a chronic condition accounting for 52% of all appointments with GPs, 65% of all hospital outpatient appointments, and 72% of hospital bed days. The NHS Improvement Plan stated that more needed to be done to support people with long-term conditions to live healthy lives and improve the responsiveness and effectiveness of health services.

This was to be achieved through support for people at three levels: self-management support for people who are able to manage their own conditions with the right advice and training; disease management by primary care teams for people with conditions that could be controlled through regular contact with a family physician, nurse, or other team members; and case management for patients with a number of conditions whose complex needs meant that they needed more intensive support than that available through self-management and disease management. Underpinning action at these three levels, the Government also highlighted the need to focus on preventing the onset of illness in the population both through the NHS and wider public policy interventions.

In 2005, came the publication of the NHS and Social Care Long-Term Conditions Model (6) as a prelude to several DH supporting documents (7–12). The Model drew explicitly on the Chronic Care Model developed by Ed Wagner and colleagues (13) and the risk stratification pyramid used in Kaiser Permanente to analyse the different levels of need experienced by the chronic care population. The inclusion of social care in the Model signified that people with chronic conditions required a range of support that extended beyond the NHS.

The importance of the NHS and social care working together was underlined in the Government's white paper, Our Health, Our Care, Our Say (14), on the future of community services. This document contained new commitments to expand the coverage of the Expert Patient Programme by 2010 by increasing enrolment to 100,000 patients. The programme focuses on the provision of generic, as opposed to disease-specific skills, and is delivered by trained lay people with experience of chronic care. An evaluation of the Programme (15) found that patients in the intervention group reported considerably greater self-efficacy and energy after 6 months compared to a control group and concluded that it was cost-effective and therefore a useful addition to existing services in the management of people with chronic conditions. In addition, disease-specific self-management programmes, such as those for people with diabetes (16, 17), offered an alternative option for some people.

Other white paper commitments were to offer personalized care plans to everyone who wanted one by 2010, establish demonstration projects to test the use of assistive technologies to help people with chronic conditions live safely at home, and to promote integrated care.

Giving people more choice over their health and social care is one of the Government's main priorities. For people with long-term conditions, choice means being given the opportunity to take more control over how they manage their condition, including support to self care, to help maintain their independence. The white paper also committed to testing a Year of Care approach to commissioning for people with long-term conditions. This approach is about ensuring commissioning of care which supports the development and delivery of individualized packages of care covering a year (or planned period of time). The individuals through their personalized care pathway should then have access to a range of choices that are evidence-based and locally available.

This year saw the publication of the government's primary and community care strategy part of the NHS Next stage Review (18, 19) lead by Lord Darzi. It has four clear themes:

- Shaping services around individuals
- Promoting healthy lives
- Continuously improving quality
- Leading local change

The strategy reiterated the importance of focusing on long-term conditions, and proposed initiatives to pilot the use of individual budgets to help people have greater control over their health and care, and to make available a Patient Prospectus to assist people understand the support available for managing a long-term condition. It also focused on primary care providers as the key to improvements in this whole policy area and described various levers and incentives to enable this to happen. It called for integrated care pilots that could enable primary health care, community health services, social care, and hospital services to work more cohesively together.

My perspective from my years in general medical practice

The 'list-based' system of general practice is widely regarded as one of the best systems of primary care in the world. Over 2 decades of accumulated evidence leads both international policy analysts and the public to their favourable conclusions of British general medical practice (20, 21). The central function of general practice is to provide care for their patients when their life events require, in the patient's eyes, professional attention. Attention that can be couched in bio-clinical and psycho-social terms reflecting the varied reasons that patients consult a trusted doctor. And the extensive training of general practitioners coupled with improved practice facilities and improved technologies means that far more extended clinical care can be delivered in primary care settings.

But there is a wider policy and management context as effective primary and community care services are at the core of a high-quality population health service, delivering important benefits if, as in the UK, the first contact by patients is almost entirely in primary care (22):

- Health outcomes are better in areas with more primary care doctors.
- People with good access to primary care are healthier than those without.

- Universal access to primary care is associated with reduced inequalities in health outcomes and the quantity and quality of primary care is associated with lower and better use of hospitals.
- Health care systems with a greater orientation towards primary care are associated with lower overall system costs.
- High-quality primary care can be as good as or better than specialised care for patients with common long term conditions and patients with co-morbidities.

Primary and community services are the setting for most people's contact with the NHS – over 90% of all contacts with the NHS take place within that setting. General Practice has arguably the key clinical role in community-based care, not least for the sheer volume of personal patient contacts that are undertaken there. GPs and nurses in general practice see more than 300 million people a year and 800,000 people a day – 80% of all the clinical consultations of the NHS.

Primary care has been defined by Professor Barbara Starfield (23) as, 'that aspect of health services that assures person focussed care over time to a defined population, accessibility to facilitate receipt of care when it is first needed, comprehensiveness of care in the sense that only rare or unusual manifestations of ill health are referred elsewhere, and coordination of care such that all facets of care (wherever received) are integrated'.

The UK general practice registered list of patients is a unique feature even amongst other first contact health care systems. It must be retained, as without it many of the attributes of general practice could not be realized. It enables better pro active care of patients who live with long-term conditions – incentivised very successfully in the Quality and Outcomes Framework of the GP contract. And is, of course, the population basis of resource allocation necessary for the policy of practice-based commissioning wherein the GP practice can voluntarily take on the budgetary responsibility for care that is delivered beyond traditional general practice.

Future policy direction is for the general practice registered population to become the population focus for extended primary and community services, giving those services a defined population responsibility '18'. A primary care 'home' with budgetary incentives to provide effective responsive services, while also focusing 'upstream'. A home for being 'the resource to its community' and in particular those living with long-term conditions. Health care is not the major contributor to health gain (23, 24). Arguably therefore, local government, as it has more influence on the broader social determinants of health, is more important than the NHS in improving the public's health. But primary health care is where bio-clinical care for the individual and addressing elements of the wider social determinants of health of the population can be brought together. For instance, 'brief interventions' by a trusted clinician within the consultation is likely to encourage and enable patients to lead healthier lives – with a supported evidence base (25). Joint working between the NHS and local government is essential at all levels and new incentives should enable such synergy. Care and case-management techniques to improve care for people with increasing severity and complexity of chronic conditions are with increasing frequency being undertaken in primary care with no lessening of quality.

But the 'new' extended primary care has some distance to go in enabling self care and self-management. Such an emphasis entails enabling health professionals to acknowledge the patient's central role in their own care, and collaborating with them to define problems, establish goals, and create treatment plans. Clinical professionals worldwide generally adopt a more didactic approach to communicating with their patients, and British doctors in primary and secondary care are generally less facilitative communicators than doctors from several other comparative countries (26–30).

Why I am not sure. Is it that the public sector lends itself well to ensuring social justice within a health care system, but creates a sense that patients should adopt the role of grateful supplicant? Are we too imbued by the concept that a want is not a need when a want should be viewed as an expressed need? Tuckett (31) described the ideal clinical consultation as being between two experts, the patient and the clinician – when expressed need can be explored. All the medical royal colleges have now incorporated self-management enablement skills in the post graduate training of doctors which portends improvement.

Conclusions

The 'new' primary care with its increased focus on long-term conditions is ideally placed to enable self care and management. Its clinicians need to ensure that patients are offered generic or specific educational courses for their chronic conditions-many are not. The quality and outcomes framework of the future could have more incentives to encourage prevention '18'. The Department of Health is to work with the National Institute of Health and Clinical Excellence to ensure there is an evidence base for such primary medical care involvement in primary prevention.

General Practice is the most trusted and popular service and so would seem ideally receptive to sharing power and to skilled facilitative patient consultations – specifically, families in poverty rate their relationship with their doctor highly (32). I feel with the new emphasis on better training, incentives within the GP contract, the altering of power relationships with the development of patient's individual budgets and patient's experiences influencing the payment of general practice, we have the building blocks to ensure more enablement to self care.

Care planning could bring so much of all this together – a manifestation of the meeting of two experts. Care plans are the product of such planning, but the process must be continual and iterative – as the former national clinical director for Diabetes at the English DH, Sue Roberts opines – the emphasis should be on the verb not the noun. Within that process, the identification of patient's educational and training needs, an agreement on where an individual budget may benefit and indeed future facilitative relationships, could all be explored.

Only time and review will tell if all these initiatives make a difference, but I feel the journey has well begun. The development of more integrated working and partnerships within the NHS and with social services and subsequently wider local government incentivised in the recent Next Stage Review Primary and Community Care Strategy '18' – with the encouragement to focus 'upstream' – also augurs well. But more fundamentally, the focus on accountability of the NHS to its patients and public not least with the development of the NHS constitution will shape and influence a change in the culture of the service. Patients and the public deserve nothing less.

References

For DH publications-website prefix- www.dh.gsi.gov.uk/ (title)

1. Department of Health (2004d) *The NHS Improvement Plan: Putting People At the Heart of Public Services.* London: HMSO.
2. *The Expert Patient: A New Approach to Chronic Disease Management for the 21st Century.* London: HMSO. http://www.dh.gov.uk/epp
3. Lorig KR., Sobel DS., et al. (1999) Evidence suggesting that a chronic disease self-management program can improve health status while reducing hospitalization: a randomized trial. *Medical Care.* 37(1): 5–14.
4. GMS contract www.nhsemployers.org or www.bma.org.uk.
5. Raising the Profile of Long Term Conditions Care. A Compendium of Information. Department of Health, 2004 and 2008. London: HMSO.
6. *Supporting People with Long Term Conditions: An NHS and Social Care Model to Support Local Innovation and Integration* (January 2005). London: HMSO.
7. Department of Health. Self Care – A Real Choice (Self Care Support – A Practical Option) (January 2005).
8. Department of Health (2005) *Public Attitudes to Self Care Baseline Survey.* Department of Health.
9. Department of Health (2005) *Supporting People with Long Term Conditions.* London: HMSO.

10. Department of Health (2005c) *The National Service Framework for Long-Term Conditions.* London: HMSO.

11. Department of Health (2006) Supporting people with long term conditions to Self Care. *A Guide to Developing Local Strategies and Good Practice.* London: Department of Health.

12. Department of Health (June 2008) *Self Care. A National View in 2007.*

13. Wagner EH., Austin BT., Davis C., et al. (2001) Improving chronic illness care: translating evidence into action. *Health Aff (Millwood).* **20**: 64–78.

14. Department of Health (2006) *Our Health, Our Care, Our Say: a New Direction for Community Services.* London: HMSO.

15. www.dh.gov.uk/en/Publicationsandstatistics/Publications/PublicationsPolicyAndGuidance/DH_080680

16. www.dafne.uk.com

17. www.desmond.org.uk

18. Department of Health (2008) *NHS Next Stage Review; Our Vision for Primary and Community Care.*

19. Department of Health (2008) *High Quality for All. NHS Next Stage Review Final Report.*

20. De Maeseneer J., Hjortdahl P., Starfield B. (June 2000) Fix what's wrong, not what's right, with general practice in Britain. *BMJ.* **320**: 1616–7.

21. Grol R., Leatherman S. (October 2002) Improving quality in British primary care: seeking the right balance. *British Journal of General Practice.* **52**(Suppl): S3–4.

22. Starfield B. (1998) *Primary Care: Balancing Health Needs, Services and Technology,* Oxford: Oxford University Press.

23. Bunker et al. (1994) Improving health; measuring effects of medical care. *The Millbank Quaterly.* **72**(2).

24. Unal B., Critchley JA., Capewell S. (2004) Explaining the decline in coronary heart disease mortality in England and Wales between 1981 and 2000. *Circulation.* **109**: 1101–7.

25. National Institute for Health and Clinical Excellence (2006) Brief interventions and referral for smoking cessation in primary care and other settings (www.publichealth.nice.org.uk).

26. Schoen C., Osborn R., Huynh PT., et al. (2005) Taking the pulse of health care systems: experiences of patients with health problems in six countries. *Health Affairs.* **WS**: 509.

27. Coulter A. (2006) *Engaging Patients in Their Healthcare: How is the UK Doing Relative to Other Countries?* Europe: Picker Institute.

28. Blakeman T., Macdonald W., Bower P., et al. (2006) A qualitative study of GPs' attitudes to self –management of chronic disease. *British Journal of General Practice.* **56**: 407–14.

29. Macdonald W., Rogers A., Blakeman T., Bower P. (2007) Practice nurses and the facilitation of self-management in primary care. *Journal of Advanced Nursing.* **62**(2): 191–9.

30. Pill R., Stott NCH., Rollnick SR., Rees M. (1998) A randomized controlled trial of an intervention designed to improve the care given in generpractice to type 2 diabetic patients: patient outcomes and professional ability to change behaviour. *Family Practice.* **15**(3): 229–35.

31. Tuckett D., Boulton M., Olsen C., Williams A. (1985) *Meetings Between Experts: An Approach to Sharing Ideas in Medical Consultations.* London: Tavistock Publications.

32. Hooper C., et al. (2007) Living with Hardship 24/7 Buttle Trust.

Chapter 9

The business case for lay-led self-management

Keith Hawley

My introduction to patient-led self-management education took place when Arthritis Care asked me to assist them in evaluating a trial of their delivery of the Arthritis Self-Management Course (ASMC) in 1996. The delivery programme seemed to me at the time to be relatively simple and straight forward. It used trained volunteers with arthritis to take a group of others through a 6-week course based on a scripted manual. This was based on research and evaluation of what people with arthritis said helped them cope best. As I listened to Jean Thompson, the trainer, and Roy Jones, the project manager, describe the results that had been achieved, I was struck with the relevance it all had to emerging agendas in health and social care. These agendas, as I perceived them as a social care professional, aimed to encourage initiatives which would foster and develop approaches to promoting peoples independence often with the intention of delaying a person's entry into residential care. Typically, the mechanisms used at that time were home care, meals on wheels, day centres, and other types of support to stay at home, which in a sense were accepting the inevitability of dependency. The ideas and practices behind self-management education excited me and seemed potentially to be offering so much more. Although not a panacea, and clearly insufficient for all people with dependency needs, it seemed to be very effective for people whose dependency was related to beliefs, self-acquired or learned, that they no longer had the ability to function without care and support from others.

Arthritis Care had noted a transformation in the functioning of many participants from their courses and how this energised a number to become active in Arthritis Care or their local communities, but they only had the funds and commitment to piloting the course in the UK. I urged them to accept responsibility for rolling the course out across the UK and believed that support from health and social services would be available to help them do so. At that time, Arthritis Care did not have the expertise to do this service development work in-house and asked me to assist. It proved to be the opportunity of a life time and working with such enthusiasts as Jean and Roy seemed to offer membership of the optimum team.

Since Arthritis Care's initial funding for the pilot phase was coming to an end, my role was to work with Jean to ensure the programme was quality assured and as cost effective and appealing to funders as possible. I then used my contacts and knowledge of the health and social care systems to approach statutory departments and explain what self-management for people with arthritis was about, how the course worked, how we ensured it was delivered as safely as possible, and how much benefit in participants we had seen and therefore how relevant it was to managers looking to develop people's capacity for self-reliance. These managers were usually officers with a responsibility for services for elderly and/or disabled people and they often responded quite well but had many competing demands for any funds available to them. Roy, who was responsible for the overall management, administration, and budgeting had an extensive network of contacts with charitable trusts and the pharmaceutical industry. It was very productive to develop partnerships with many from these fields too, and ultimately this assisted us to consolidate our funding and secure technical support in the fields of Public Relations and Communications, without which I doubt that we could have influenced government and commissioners to the extent we did.

We did not actually ask for any funding from statutory sources until we were satisfied that we had a robust system for ensuring quality in place, had honed the programme content and decided on the delivery concepts to the point where we could have confidence that we were able to deliver with equal effectiveness and consistency throughout the UK. Since we had little real local infrastructure in place, we needed to take a project development approach. This entailed targeting areas where, based on knowledge about need and enthusiasm for development on the part of Arthritis Care's local networks, development could be envisaged if resources could be found. We then asked for sufficient funds to enable Arthritis Care to appoint a local leader, known as a Self-Management Trainer (SMT) who would help recruit, train, deploy, and support a team of volunteer tutors and course arrangers. Usually, this was to be a team of around 12 with an expectation that they would build up to delivering 8 courses per year. We figured at that time, late 1990s, that this local delivery capacity could then continue to offer courses if we could raise about £2,500 per course. The local delivery teams where managed through the SMTs by Jean Thompson from Central Office and very ably supported by her administrative assistant, Lisa who was constantly on the telephone sorting out queries about manuals, books, expenses, venues, but most importantly conveying to the SMTs and the volunteers that they were valued and their issues were taken seriously. The local delivery teams also related to Arthritis Cares development officers who provided general services and support to the extensive branch network. It was their job to try and integrate the self-management courses into Arthritis Care's other works and help the SMTs develop capacity and recruit participants.

The biggest challenge initially was making the case for funding to health and social care professionals who may have had little or no experience of self-management education for people with long-term conditions and were stuck in a mind set of delivering more of the type of services they were familiar with. There were also issues of how professionals saw their responsibilities and how we managed the fact that health care professionals tended to focus on disease, while social services' concerns were more on loss of capacity. It was not very effective, for example, asking social services to provide funding for a service for people with arthritis, since the immediate reaction was that arthritis was a medical condition and the responsibility of health. On the other hand, if we asked for funds to assist people with a functional impairment to overcome and restore a degree of independence, we could almost certainly guarantee ourselves a hearing. Similarly, asking health for funding to promote independence would not move many funders unless it could be linked to an argument that costs would be saved elsewhere in the health care budget. Even then, it might be suggested that 'it should really be social services'. It was fortunate, therefore that at that time a specific fund had been established to encourage health and social care works together better. This was known as Joint Funding and it proved ideal for our purposes since we were able to argue that, although the person's condition was arthritis, clearly a health issue, the challenge to them was dealing with the constraints it placed on their ability to function, which is a social services responsibility. Attending a self-management course offered something that both health and social services could latch on to. On the one hand, it helped people live better with their condition helping to reduce pain without drugs and on the other, it enabled them to regain some independence, possibly removing their needs for direct services. We were greatly assisted in our arguments by several studies on the impact of the ASMC or as it was re-branded, 'Challenging Arthritis', which suggested that, as a result of participating in a course, people achieved, better pain management, reduction in depression, positive beliefs about their abilities to control the effects of arthritis, and a reduction in visits to GPs.

Although we sought and needed to convince health and social care professionals that investing in self-management for people with arthritis was supportive to the policy frameworks in which they operated, we also appealed to them to see the intrinsic benefits of it for people living with a long-term condition. We wanted the professionals to recognize that helping people to become empowered was a good end in itself, particularly when it enabled them to become part of a mobilization of community resources and enabled people usually seen as 'patients' or 'clients' to become resources in themselves. We were delighted when some professionals became as excited about this as we were.

The approach we took to raising funds was very successful and generated considerable interest in 'lay-led' self-management which professionals quickly saw could have application to a much wider group than those with arthritis. Indeed, somewhat to our bemusement, some statutory agencies took the view that it would be inequitable to fund a programme that only benefited people with arthritis and suggested that we should come back when we had a programme that would benefit a wider group of people with long-term conditions. It seemed a bit like saying they would not fund hip operations because they only benefitted people with a hip problem. In fact, Arthritis Care did have access to a generic programme for people with a broad range of conditions. This had been developed at Stanford as a follow-up to the arthritis course, and Jean Thompson was qualified to train the leadership staff to deliver it. However, Arthritis Care was not then in a position to deliver it themselves alongside the arthritis course for various reasons related to mission and capacity. It was timely and fortunate, therefore, that the Long-Term Medical Conditions Alliance (LMCA) decided to look at self-management for people across the range of conditions and asked for Arthritis Care's help to develop capacity in other patient organizations to deliver the generic Chronic Disease Self-Management Course (CDSMC).

The partnership between Arthritis Care and LMCA was a productive one. It led to around eight patient organizations starting to develop as providers of self-management and working together to build upon the quality assurance system developed by Arthritis Care. These organizations were mainly bodies that had a mission for supporting people with a specific condition. They had an intimate understanding of the needs of people with that condition and it was significant that most of them were willing to pilot a generic course, often with a generic group of participants, although some delivered only to their particular condition group. Considerable enthusiasm was generated and there was, briefly as it sadly turned out to be, a period of rapid development of capacity across the country through these organizations, funded by Social Services, Health Organizations, Trusts, Patient Organizations themselves and Pharmaceutical Companies.

It was sound, value-grounded development using principles of patient involvement, management, and empowerment, focussing entirely on achieving benefits for those involved. It increased their sense of taking control while giving them space and opportunity limited only by the will and capacity that they had to achieve and not what others sought to impose upon them. How did this work in practice?

The patient organizations were usually able to recruit participants through their own networks, and we found that people who were recruited to a self-management course had often become bogged down by their condition. They may have felt victimized by it and almost certainly were overwhelmed by the restrictions it placed on them in going about their daily lives. People, who may previously have had responsible well-paid jobs through which they earned respect and self-esteem, had become infantilized through their dependence on health care professionals and others who could often offer little beyond medication and information leaflets. Attending a course gave the participants an opportunity to challenge this superimposed self-image, and acquire skills to put themselves back in the driving seat of their lives. At the end of each course, therefore there could be 10 people who were not going to take everything simply as offered to them. They were going to ask questions and those questions were going to make those to whom the questions were addressed, reflect on both the questions and their answers. Often those questioned would be health care professionals, officers in organizations they were members of, etc. Of the 10 'graduates', some might want to do more than live their own lives, they would want to make a difference to others. These often became tutors, contributed to the programme in some other way or became activists in the patient organization who had sponsored the course they attended. The energy developed in an individual through attending a course thus permeated through the programme, producing a constant stream of new tutors, some of whom went on to become trainers or managers in the programme. The programmes thrived as a result and a unique camaraderie developed amongst tutors, programme organizers and the sponsoring organizations, based on an awareness that they were making a real difference to the lives of people living with a long-term condition. These in turn were trying to make a difference in the patient bodies that represented them, to those who provided them with services, to their families, and to the wider social and economic environment where they lived. It would be an exaggeration to describe this as a 'movement', but we certainly saw something that, although often not devoid of tensions, was exciting and wanted to tell the world about it.

The Department of Health listened, and the work was mentioned positively in the 1999 white paper on public health which said that the government would be setting up an 'Expert Patient Task Force' to consider how it could be given wider backing. It was interesting that the DH focused on the 'Expert Patient' aspects of self-management education since Roy Jones who was so instrumental in the early work at Arthritis Care, had sometimes referred to lay-led self-management as giving recognition to the fact that patients coping with a long-term condition are often the experts at dealing with its consequences and that the courses enable them to share their expertise with others. As a result of the task force, the government invested substantially in an 'Expert Patients Programme'. This did not take the form of feeding needed resources into the pioneering patient organizations, but entailed the establishment of a new training and development organization to evolve a separate provider network based on PCTs. This caused dismay in many of the pioneering organizations who had hoped funds would be fed their way to sustain and build on the developments that had inspired government thinking. They also, and justifiably as it turned out, feared for the continuation of their existing statutory income streams given that PCTs were to be given incentives to develop their own programmes.

It might be concluded that if the DH had made such a significant commitment to establishing self-management education across England, the business case had been made. This was not so. Many PCTs were not convinced by what they were being asked to do and neither were all the doctors, nurses, and other health care professionals directly in contact with patients. Some of these professionals believed that they were already delivering self-management education to patients. The fact that many Expert Patients Programmes in the PCTs were positioned in departments dealing with public and patient involvement and liaison, rather than clinical issues, also tended to distort the message. There was a danger that self-management education would be seen as being about developing advocates and reformers rather than offering an opportunity to patients who, with better self-management skills might, just might, want to go on to be advocates and reformers. Distortion of the real purpose of self-management education has been a continuing issue. Because it can lead to so many good outcomes, people going back into full-time education or work, becoming community activists and so on – organizations and professionals with an interest in fostering these outcomes have often seized on self-management education as a way of achieving their objectives. Similarly, health and social care finance managers have seen it has a possible way of reducing hospital admissions, medication budgets, home care costs, and contact time with professionals. Self-management education does of course achieve all these objectives, but not all the time and not for everyone who participates in a course. Achieving these outcomes is not its starting point. What it universally achieves is what it was intended to achieve by its authors: happier, better motivated people who feel more in control of their lives while living with a long-term condition, and better able to manage and make choices. The pioneering patient organizations saw this very clearly. It was their focus and it was sufficient for them. Funding was sought simply as a means of providing more of it rather than as a cash payment to enable a purchasing organization achieve its targets. With a few notable exceptions however, delivery of lay-led self-management in England has moved away from the patient organizations, and the current generation of providers, whether in the PCTs or third sector, are likely to be very significantly dependent financially on the decisions of commissioners. These, as purchasers, will be driven by considerations of how far self-management education enables them to meet their commissioning objectives and targets and what value for money against alternatives it offers. In short, they will be taking commercially orientated decisions and may demand services that in terms of content, quality, and cost match specifications they determine rather than those considered more appropriate by the provider. It is unclear what this means for self-management and especially lay-led self-management. Could it mean a worrying shift for lay-led self-management's very raison d'être from the achievement of life changing benefit and empowerment for an individual, to its utility in supporting the achievement of the aims of organizations unaware of, or unmoved by, its creators and developers view of its intrinsic value?

Chapter 10

Implementing pilot EPP within the wider strategy to support self care

An interview with Ayesha Dost

Policy Adviser, Department of Health 1995–2008[1]

Roy Jones: Prior to managing EPP pilot, how long had you been aware of the Stanford courses?
Ayesha Dost: In 1995, I was writing a paper for the Department of Health on health futures focussing on futuristic approaches, some technical and some common sense methodologies that became *Foresight in Health.* Having worked on similar concerns for over two decades, I had realized the need to inject new ideas into some of the archaic governmental systems in the UK. For example, social models of care were not commonplace in the health and social care statutory sector. There were some useful local initiatives such as for people with diabetes and back pain, but these had not yet been evaluated. I drew on my experience in India. *Foresight* mentioned the specific self care skills needed by people with long-term conditions and referred to Kate Lorig's work which was attractive because it had been evaluated and provided evidence on the efficacy of interventions closer to the home. Self care support was subsequently identified as a social model of care and a practical option that could be provided in any care setting, community, or statutory.

RJ: Some Australian work described the Stanford research quality as grade B but its importance as grade A. What did the department learn from early involvement with self care and self-management?
AD: Even today, I don't think there is much better than grade B worldwide. In the UK, evaluations in the 1990s were not robust as the sample size was small due to the overall programme itself having been delivered to only a few people. Also, academics have their own self-imposed limitations as they apply research methods relevant for drug trials to social models of care.

Researchers from different countries tend not to arrive at common robust methodologies on how to assess outcomes of social models. International perspectives are needed on crucial outcomes such as the building up of social capital.

However, just as with NHS Direct, we learnt that sometimes there are policies we need to implement even where the evidence is patchy. From work in several countries, including among people with leprosy in India, I knew self care skills training crucially enabled people to take care of their health as well as fulfil their aspirations, and we could not ignore that just because the evidence was incomplete. You have to learn by doing, and by doing we would also gather the evidence.

RJ: Tell me about the CMO, Sir Liam Donaldson's term the 'expert patient'.
AD: For many years, focus was on hospital care, but now in order for 'person centred care' to be implemented, we were developing services 'outside the hospital' and closer to home. The CMO agreed that self care skills training would help the patient become an expert at taking care of their life and health, and the term expert patient was coined; in other words, individuals would become expert at having patience, not simply experts of their ailments.

RJ: Do you think Sir Liam and practitioners shared an understanding of the term 'expert patient'? Or, was there some confusion?
AD: Sir Liam didn't get involved in the day-to-day activities of EPP, but some health professionals may have defined expertise as medical ability rather than self care. Actually, EPP participants became expert in having patience! This is a real ability that the course brings about. In Islam, patience is called *sabr*, a most important quality. Having *sabr* means being the best possible human being. I think the term, 'expert patient' is quite appropriate. What we're talking about is people finding their hidden depths. It is the expertise in self care. I am sure Sir Liam wanted expert patients and professionals to partner and not compete with one another. It must be understood that while people do self care, it is professionals who have to support self care, meaning that professionals have a role to play in supporting patients become the experts they can be.

RJ: In the introduction to the EP report he talks about patients knowing more about their condition than their doctors.
AD: This is true too. We cannot ignore the technical knowledge that patients develop. There are several components to the term 'expert patients'. The key 'organic' component is:

> These individuals will have patience, high self-esteem, self-efficacy, skills to self care and ability to value themselves. As these individuals willingly network with one

another social capital builds up. And this is what creates a vibrant society which feels human, respects 'the other', and is not a 'mutual' interest society. I don't continue to participate in this programme because I want help from others. I do it because it is a human thing to do. It is a way of being.

The other top four components are more mechanistic, Expert patients have:

- Knowledge and information; sometimes this may exceed that of the professionals, but it is there for shared decision making and not to threaten.
- Skills to use technology and devices that are available for disease specific or general needs.
- Skills to use the available information.
- Skills to become part of a wider network for active participation in a thriving society. And this is not about being there *for*; it is about *belonging* to.

This is who expert patients are. It is doable and requires that health and social care professionals understand and support this approach. It is interesting that Long-Term Conditions Alliance (LMCA) and other players in self-management did not maintain proper registers of those who had participated in their courses; the registers would have given a huge impetus for social capital to build up.

RJ: Tell me about the idea that every Primary Care Trust (PCT) should have the opportunity to try out EPP.
AD: The department must provide equal access to care services for all across the country. The fact that we may face challenges in implementing social models of care does not mean that we should not attempt to make them available in all PCT areas.

RJ: Do you think we should have done more with health professionals to get them on board EPP?
AD: I have heard comments that the term 'expert patients' minimizes the skills of health professionals and diminishes them in stature. This is nonsense. The NHS has highly qualified professionals who are not going to feel threatened by patients who may be well informed or aware of their conditions! On the contrary, many would love to have the opportunity to talk to confident patients who are able to co-create good health. However, EPP was not like a new medicine where professionals draw on biochemistry studies to understand its efficacy. The 'social model of care' calls for a paradigm shift and while the word 'expert' does not create a contentious issue, professionals may need to accept less robust evidence to appreciate the valuable difference that self care support can make to the lives and health of people. It is however encouraging seeing

programmes like EPP becoming part of NHS vocabulary and are slowly but surely here to stay regardless of what the future of the EPP CIC might be.

RJ: Is it about looking at things from a different viewpoint?
AD: Yes, it is about making a connection. Health professionals do not readily connect improving services for patients with EPP courses or with self care support. When patients keep returning and you recognize they need some upskilling and you don't know how to do it, then we need to somehow ensure that professionals make the connection. It is easy after that because substantial provision of self care support services is already out there.

RJ: I was impressed by the quality of people who applied for staff positions in the EPP pilot. All candidates met professional standards and had personal experience of a long-term condition. NHS human resources found this unusual.
AD: Yes, and the candidates became a hugely skilled resource for the programme. It was also an opportunity for the new members of staff to upgrade their skills. We discovered that despite years of experience of a condition, sometimes they lacked confidence due to their relationship to the condition as well as a dependency on health professionals.

Whereas in acute illness the professional is in command, for long-term conditions either a partnership with the professional is required or the patient needs to be much more in command. Both the NHS and the individual need to accept that the latter is the biggest resource for the care system.

RJ: When KL was initially talking to people with arthritis she found a large resource of problem solving skill.
AD: A long-term condition can make you helpless or bring out the best in you. By being dependent on them, health professionals can make you worse than you already feel given your condition, or they can upskill you by making available self care skills training. It is obvious that you will choose to be an asset to society rather than feel a burden on it.

RJ: The DH was generating new initiatives for caring for people with long-term conditions. Do you think Expert Patients keyed into those initiatives sufficiently?
AD: There was a clear agenda for the care of people with long-term conditions. In fact, way back in 1999 as a prelude to the NHS Plan we had our own 'care pyramid strategy' (also borrowed from us by the Scottish Executive and the Australians), which some stakeholders brought back to us calling it 'Kaiser pyramid'!! Quite a farce; some people prefer American labels! Others were

inclined to see CDSMC as one size fits all. But, we had already arrived at an understanding that we needed a wider self care *support* strategy of which self care skills training formed one part and within which CDSMC one component. The wider strategy ensured provision of self care information, devices, technologies, and peer networks. EPP itself went beyond CDSMC by making it a nation-wide NHS programme and addressing the issue of bringing EPP participants together as a national resource. The skills training course under the Working in Partnership Programme is another component of the wider self care support strategy. NHS Direct provides self care information.

RJ: So, what did DH learn from all this?

AD: EPP was made equally accessible to all groups of people by providing it under the NHS. At its height, we had 28 centres across the country with courses in ten languages. We now have the UK evidence that self care skills training can lead to beneficial outcomes for patients as well as the care system. Another lesson was that the trained EPP participants, volunteer tutors, and paid trainers wanted to keep in close contact with one another, which meant that a supported effort could prevent a national resource from dispersing and help create social capital on an unprecedented scale.

RJ: The idea of starting a new venture with a wholly new structure loads a great deal on the individuals involved.

AD: The EPP has now moved outside the NHS and offers courses to commissioners willing to purchase them. To function as a business model keeping cost of courses low, is a challenge even if a self-imposed one! It can still work but only if it is a two tier system having at one level a small core national resource responsible for quality, keeping periodic assessments of tutors and trainers simple and not overly bureaucratic. Costly expenditure on quality assurance must be watched. Social models of care do not require heavy handed costly quality checks. The second tier would be essentially local with energetic involvement of local community organizations in training volunteer tutors, keeping them together through self-organized activities.

Ideally, the social capital would be best nurtured through healthy partnerships with local bodies such as PCTs, social services, GP surgeries or community, and voluntary organizations as they already carry out public health, community care, and/or public involvement functions. Also, DH targets can only be met if the number of volunteer tutors grows. That can happen only through local engagement and partnerships.

Despite new arrangements, it may still be useful to associate the NHS brand with EPP. I hope commissioners of EPP services, whether they are NHS public health managers or private sector employers, will use the NHS logo if it gives participants more confidence. The Stanford license would in fact be available free under DH agreement if used under an NHS banner for NHS patients.

RJ: You were keen to see disease-specific modules.
AD: We found from participant feedback that there was a great demand for information about people's own conditions. That meant that people were now ready to utilize information and were actively seeking it from us. The idea was that after completing the 6-week course, participants from a number of courses within a PCT could come together for a seventh-week module in disease-specific groups. These would be supported by local health professionals in a partnership style. Sadly, this partnership element somehow got left out as the EPP progressed.

RJ: You were keen on participation of the voluntary sector.
AD: I wanted voluntary and community agencies to become active partners in EPP. For LMCA, however, it was all or nothing. The LMCA wanted to manage EPP, but that was not practical as their outfit was considered undersized for handling such a large programme. They had limited experience of running a few small sized projects. Moreover, the roll out of EPP could not be delayed given the CMO's timeframe, and there was pressure to get on with implementation. LMCA and other voluntary agencies could have sent their member patients and volunteers for training via local PCTs creating a much larger pool of participants and tutors, but this did not happen. Only a few organizations participated very unfortunately.

RJ: You said you had discussions with the Scottish Executive.
AD: I made two presentations to the Scottish Executive and contributed to the NHS24 strategy and national framework document they brought out. Self care support is now well entrenched in Scottish health policies and programmes including NHS24.

RJ: You once said getting the terminology and language right was very important.
AD: Language can set the direction of travel. The phrase self-management became popular in USA. In the Department, we felt that this term was limited, had a commercial ring, and seemed more to do with being efficient. We were developing self care as one of the pillars of the NHS alongside primary care, intermediate care, secondary care, and social care, so that professionals and practitioners see it as a key component of the care system and therefore gear themselves to support self care in a system in which people would also play a

strong partnership role. Also, for many, self-management had come to mean management of symptoms, whereas we were proposing to support people by enhancing their self care skills as a way of being human with respect for oneself and others.

RJ: *So, self care includes making time for children, not beating yourself up over things you cannot do …?*
AD: Self care is more than looking after yourself. It is about creating an atmosphere in your home, in local communities, in the wider system. The word 'care' is important. We care for life; we care for humanity, etc. The term management is not entirely negative, but it can be limiting.

RJ: *What have you learned as a professional with a long term condition?*
AD: For a self care support programme to succeed, each player must grasp the self care terminology, where care and self are both key words, and those who provide support must have the right intention. A humble approach has to be modelled by the leaders and trainers. If you do not care and are arrogant when leading your staff or role modelling or training people, the whole programme is endangered. Some senior EPP staff had technical knowledge but lacked role modelling or leadership qualities. The EPP culture and ethos were affected by this, creating some unhappiness and as the evaluation shows, outcomes varied in different EPP regions. The very nature of the programme was to be support-ive and to generate laughter and feeling of joy, most of all for staff themselves. Instead of being fully involved, if even one junior staff or one course partici-pant feels disempowered, the very basis of the programme is shaken.

RJ: *Any other lessons …?*
AD: People need to maintain the skills they have learnt through networks which are self-organized and sustainable, with the system putting certain support mechanisms in place for them.

RJ: *What particular insight would you offer the government?*
AD: To further raise professional awareness of social models of care. And to enhance the skills of professionals in supporting self care. So, the key message for the government is: professionals must be trained in the concept of self care early on.

RJ: *This is such a different paradigm to the introduction of new medicines.*
AD: Absolutely. Investment in people is cumulative rather than repetitive (as with antibiotics). Every time a patient is treated, a medicine is prescribed which

is consumed and disappears with the illness, and has to be repeated if illness re-emerges. When self care support and training is provided to individuals, the skills or networks can stay with them and are even further passed on as the trained individual trains or connects others among the family, friends, or community. This process is cumulative. Unfortunately, researchers usually measure linear benefits of interventions rather than accrued gains!!

RJ: At the outset, we thought it worthwhile to evolve an NHS structure for supporting self care.
AD: I have provided some research evidence on DH self care website in addition to evaluation of EPP. It is important that research on social models looks at process outcomes such as cumulative and multiplicative build up of social capital and their impact on the self, and further whether the consequence might be the creation of an active society of engaged citizens. We need evidence on implications for our unique NHS system. We need also to see the comparability and complementarities between a range of our initiatives, such as WiPP, NHS Direct, NHS24, EPP, back pain, and diabetes specific solutions, online programmes, and many others. When you consider all these together, it is an amazing rich picture!! The NHS must now harness its resource of 15.4 million people with long-term conditions!

Speaking of our joint thinking on evolving a structure befitting the NHS, one crucial point is that the single factor in the success of the programme to support self care has been your contributions in terms of its initial development through to its successful implementation. Your vision (that we shared way back in 1996), conceptual clarity, and the deep empathy you generally have for people not only got the programme going but also helped shape it to become an internationally enviable approach in the care of people with long-term conditions. I will always remember those animated discussions we had, initially you, Jim Phillips and I, and sometimes Keith Hawley. All of us were very good together. I would like here to express to you my gratitude and many felicitations.

Endnotes

1 Interviews were recorded at editor's home (December 2007) and King's Fund, London (January 2008).

Chapter 11

Self-management and patient and public involvement

An Interview with Bob Sang

Roy Jones: Tell me about the Stanford Programmes and Patient and Public involvement.

Bob Sang: Some years ago (2001), I saw the emergence of different modes of public patient involvement and one of these, a key plank, was self-management for people with long-term conditions. When I published a piece in the Health Services Journal, Judy Wilson rang to thank me for highlighting this work. Of course, my introduction to the whole endeavour of bringing the Chronic Disease Self-Management Course into the NHS started with a conversation with one Roy Jones.

RJ: I didn't know that.

BS: You invited me to Arthritis Care to meet Richard Gutch and colleagues. Self-management made immediate sense for two reasons. First, it connected with my experience of working in partnership with the advocacy movement for people with learning disabilities. The principle was that these people could have, with proper support, a voice and a big say in the development of the services they used. The other reason was because, in pioneering advocacy developments, we would not have made progress without the active support of people in the service who 'got it', and were prepared to risk engaging with this kind of social innovation. For me, the CDSMC is a social innovation.

RJ: Starting in Arthritis Care we were naturally focused on people with arthritis. Our sense was that often, these were oppressed people, bottled up inside a medical model.

BS: The first people to challenge the medical model were people with learning disabilities and their supporters. Of course, if you're born with a learning disability, you're not thick, but to be incarcerated in institutions with pre-scribed regimens for all of your life was really, particularly from a civil liberties perspective, not on. But the strength and power of those people meant we had leverage after the dreadful hospital scandals of the 1970s. Other people in the late 70s challenging the medical model, were the mental health users in the anti-psychiatry movement. There was a need for a different model that allowed people to establish purposes outside of being a patient. We saw people at Arthritis Care able to break free and reflect on their lives in terms of their wider roles, aspirations, and ambitions. That has become a thing for me ... people don't have needs, they have ambitions.

RJ: That was found in some of Malcolm Battersby's work in Australia. Even people with psychotic conditions have things they want to achieve.
BS: I must challenge you: you're still using the word *even*. As it happens, living most of my adult life with depression, I can say it has become a resource for me. I can tell when it is coming on. When I learnt self-management through the educational route, it was a fantastic release and that too provided a resonance for me. I saw self-management and self-managed learning happening inside the pilot EPP, Challenging Arthritis and Living with Long-term Illness groups. When they discovered confidence they asked, 'What shall I do with this?' Some people chose to get on with their lives, 'I have served this disease long enough!' Others wanted to contribute, train as a tutor, seek roles in the voluntary sector, or contribute to the re-planning of services (commissioning in the modern jargon).

RJ: Would you see that as a rediscovery of self?
BS: That's a really good way of putting it. Self-managed learning gives you the skills to engage reflectively and rediscover yourself, make adjustments and also evaluate your skills and qualities. I have tremendous dialogues with clinicians reflecting on their practice and struggles with complexity. They often need a sounding board and most do not have the skills of self-managed learning. They have neither mentors nor proper supervision. So, I bring that skill set into a context where it is needed saying I am here to help learning, not I am someone with experience as a patient.

RJ: Many 'course graduates' have had similar experience.
BS: Doctors have their own peer-group pressures but they can change very quickly once they attain critical mass. There has been a lot of rhetoric about patients as super-consumers selecting material from the Internet. That information is completely useless if the people haven't got self-management skills and the confidence that goes with it. They may end up in a destructive or collusive debate with a clinician or anything in between, but it does not enrich the learning.

People have habits of learning from an education system that's been histori- cally didactic. Consequently, they're often too uncritical of information seen as coming from a higher authority; or fear and anxiety drives them to hear what they want to hear. Patient involvement work, in some ways, is very like being a tutor in a self-management programme, you learn to facilitate, to give people the opportunity to develop a sufficient sense of security and confidence in the group's process so that they can have their own beliefs and assumptions challenged, begin to take on new ones, rediscover talents within, reawaken ambition, etc.

RJ: Let's go back to that period around 2000/2001 for a moment. At that time, the CMO, Sir Liam Donaldson, was finishing work on the Expert Patients Report.
BS: The first time I saw Sir Liam in action was at the launch conference for the Expert Patient Programme (EPP). The 2 years of financial stringency after the Labour government came in were over and in 1998/1999 the reform agenda was launched. We had the NHS Plan, etc., but the rhetoric was also about improving choice and improving the quality and safety of services. Sir Liam said, 'This will need a paradigm shift but in the end it will not be managers of doctors that lead the shift but patients'. He spoke with utter conviction about the work that had been developed at Stanford, its significance and the opportunity created by developing the EPP pilot. I don't know where that conviction came from, but basically I think he trusted Kate Lorig's work when he'd met her.

I met Kate in 2002 when on a study group to the US that involved the then health minister Hazel Blears. This initiative was kept in DH's public health section not the NHS. That is really important; it meant Ayesha Dost and her colleagues were in a line of reporting to Sir Liam, not to the Chief Executive of the NHS.

From a public health leader point of view, Sir Liam saw a methodology that engaged people in managing their own health improvement: the very people most likely to generate increased demand in the NHS. For those of us rooted in community-based pubic health, this made complete sense, both in personal and economic terms. By now, Derek Wanless had been commissioned by Gordon Brown to look at how you could sustain the system. Wanless talked about the 'fully engaged scenario' and to be blunt, I think self-management support was seen as one of the keys for a sustainable NHS. Then we ran into the problem of evaluation and of criteria set out in a medical research rather then a social policy research model. It was a problem.

Let's divert for a moment. If you think the job of the NHS is to treat lots of people in a curative model, that's fine but it's not sustainable with an ageing population, improving medical knowledge leading to improving diagnostics, and growing treatment options. It will drown in activity and increasing specialization. However, if the job is to sustain and enhance the resilience of people in communities, then you are looking for different models and different measures. If people are looking at measuring clinical outcomes for the EPP and not at measures of improved personal and group resilience and contribution to social capital, then for me, they are missing the point.

RJ: And missing that evaluation of public engagement and public resilience, the temptation is to focus on evaluating medical outcomes from courses.
BS: Let's take a tutor's example where you might say there has been no benefit at all. Someone came and for 5 weeks said nothing, preferring to sit in a corner. At the end of the final session, he said, 'Thank you. This has been great. I feel so much better about my condition now. I can get on with my life'. No measurable clinical benefit was apparent. We forget the literature on preferred learning styles. 'Quiet reflectors' are one part of that mix. It is necessary to respect people's preferred styles just like preferences around food and drink.

RJ: My grandchildren go to a junior school where they are streamed by preferred learning styles.
BS: That's right and it goes back to engagement. People are discovering that the key issue for running a successful school is to spot when children are disengaging and find out what is happening. It is not the children: they are not the problem. Children want to learn and they need to reconnect. For me engagement and learning go hand in hand. Something grabs people's passion and their interest.

RJ: Moving on … So much had been learned. Arthritis Care was enlarging capacity by taking on the CDSMC. The pilot phase of the EPP is coming to an end and you convene a day's discussion in Portland Place.
BS: My role is that of a friend, catalyst, and supporter with special links to the patient/public engagement agenda. One product of those discussions was Co-Creating Health because Stephen Thornton, the CEO of the Health Foundation, came and discerned something important. What cracked it for many people was the growing recognition (culminating in the publication of *Our Health, Our Care, Our Say*), that 80–85% of the activity in the NHS is generated by about 10% of the population. If you proactively and collaboratively manage long-term conditions and disabilities, that is where you have the best possibility of improving the quality of outcomes of sustaining a publicly funded health and social care system. In the renal field, if you can work

proactively with people with early signs of hypertension, vascular disease, diabetes, etc., you can prevent numbers of people coming through to end stage renal disease. Those people cost hugely more than their personal budgets.

We are getting some recognition among commissioning chief executives who see that if they don't get to grips with the co-morbid population, then they will drown in activity. They have good reason for viewing self-management programmes as necessary enhancements to traditional clinical services.

RJ: As the EPP pilot came towards its end we had this amazing body of people, an excellent staff, deployed across England. Where are they going to go? The Community Interest Company (CIC) emerges. Have you any idea where it came from?

BS: I had a little responsibility here because I was part of the original team that wrote the paper promoting the idea of social enterprise. Hazel Blears, then a health minister, led a group that visited Stanford and Chicago, where on South Side (in Barack Obama country), we saw them developing social enterprise structures. We reckoned 5 things were needed to grow a local health economy from the ground up

- Self-management
- Access to appropriate lay advocacy
- Citizen, lay leadership
- Social enterprise
- Collaboration with a multi-professional team

If you had all of those things in one locality, then it could begin to grow *health improvement* as a collaborative endeavour.

RJ: But South Side has a culture and identity of its own. Moving from there to creating a <u>national</u> community interest company is a big leap.

BS: Correct. When I reported on the CIC-based focus groups round the country. I found tutors recognized what Patricia Greenhalgh's recent analysis in the British Medical Journal also demonstrates, namely the need to grow on the ground, what I call a community engagement model of developing self-management. I have also started to think of this as a social co-production model – nurturing the core economy; the work that is done outside the market. In other words, what we identified as potential transferable learning going to Chicago and meeting Kate in San Francisco has actually been validated by Trish's analysis. This goes way beyond some of the critiques that have come from people who have taken a rather narrow evaluation paradigm. Experienced tutors and senior trainers were already working in a community engagement model taking issues like health inequalities seriously and innovating at ground level. They understood community engagement because they had to. Part of the participant recruitment is reaching out; using networks of organizations and recognizing that people live fairly atomistic lives, but networks can reach disadvantaged groups. One of the unfair criticisms of the EPP is that it is middle class. This is rubbish. Given half a chance, all sort of people quickly connect and join the new networks.

The trouble with the CIC model, (a community interest company), is that it over emphasises *company* at the expense of *community interest*. If the business model involves running a centralized training organization with a standardized product and achieving sales volume, then all the community engagement stuff is irrelevant. If you're a networked learning organization and your main resource is a network of lay leaders, building an infrastructure that fits the community and the neighbourhood, and that is the kind of people I met, then there is a serious disconnect with the emerging business model of the EPP–CIC. The reason was probably very straightforward. The government needed a funding mechanism to keep the whole thing going and they attached a sales target to it. The other issue that causes tension is that they have gone away from the ethos of the way the EPP was grown by its original leaders.

I predict there will be a crisis in the next year because the business model is not sustainable given the need for a throughput of 100,000 people a year. It cannot be done on the current model. There are also issues with the US partners running the online training. In fancy academic terms, there has been over commoditization of the EPP and it's based on a sales/business model. The CIC is a holding board and organization with a centralist operational model and it will increasingly become detached from the people in the field.

RJ: Meanwhile work has been building up in the Health Foundation's Co-Creating Health (CCH) project.
BS: I cannot comment too much. I can say it is working well in patches. But partnerships have to be based on shared values and clarity of purpose. To be fair to the people running that programme, the NHS is going through so much managerial/structural change that people do not have the space to develop the relationships that can bear the level of trust needed to sustain this level of co-creativity.

It is important to reflect on the UK context.

First, there are three things that an NHS chief executive could get sacked for:

- Financial balance
- Waiting time targets, both in emergency care and planned care
- Any increase in hospital acquired infections on their patch

Other priorities get obscured with the consequence that their job is seen as managing acute medicine.

Second, in terms of what is happening with the professions, physicians are struggling to establish their position because the surgical model drives much of this. Some physicians are emerging with a holistic model, but only when this paradigm is established in the medical mind set do you find tolerance, not just for self-management, but co-creation, integrated medicine and the use of effective alternatives such as acupuncture for back pain. (It's interesting that NICE has recently produced guidance supporting the use of acupuncture for people with back pain in the month of Bob's death.)

Third, is the way clinician time is accounted. GPs with their Quality and Outcome Frameworks (QOFs) and the way the system incentivised on throughput is *not* on a relationship-based model of care. The way reform along with structural change has gone has not only broken up relationships, but also limited the time to relate. When I talk to GPs about engagement I say, rather than seeing people with arthritis, say, in a way that looks like uncontrollable demand, why not start running group sessions about managing pain, with a bit of skilled facilitation? Bring in the pain consultant as an advisor to your programme. Twenty people are allowed 8 min each in consultation time, and let's say two meetings. That's 160 minutes!

RJ: In groups you can cut this to 2 hours and still do pretty well.
BS: Absolutely right! You've got it. What they need, and this is where I think they're missing a trick, are some of the skills of facilitation and group working, and the process of supporting self-management.

RJ: OK. Let's close by talking about commissioning.
BS: Commissioning is about solving complex problems. People often say about patient involvement, 'Ah! But they are not representative.' You can do all your sampling, surveys, and analyses, but you also need to recruit from the growing pool that has learned peer learning through self-management: they can help you solve them. As a professional facilitator, I put people through a peer learning process. They do not behave like stakeholders in a managed group. I have a wonderful time with some of these skilled patients in the room. They add so much value. The doctors say, 'This is good! We get to agreement much faster than when we're just on our own'. (The doctors never agree on their own partly because one of the hidden truths is that medical evidence supporting service change is usually contentious.) Balancing safety, fair access, and what can be afforded is a complex task and experienced patients get it, just like that! They become, not heated campaigners but bringers of light and insight and simplicity.

This is my challenge to managers about having atypical patients. I say, 'You wouldn't like it if I called you typical managers would you?' And nobody wants to be. 'So why think there's a typical patient?' They want to be valued because of their experience, their track record and the fact they are willing to learn and share.

RJ: Thank you Bob we really needed this contribution and perspective.

This chapter is edited from the transcript of an interview recorded on 2nd June 2009. Bob died suddenly 3 days later.

Chapter 12

The Expert Patients Programme – Community Interest Company: The future

Simon Knighton

So, how do you take an established, successful programme out of the NHS and turn it into a sustainable business? I joined EPP–CIC as Chief Executive in June 2007. It had been up and running since April 2007 and it was my task, along with the board, to turn the growing interest in the programme into a business that could not only provide a much-valued service to millions of people living with long-term health conditions (LTCs) but also be financially sustainable for the long term.

The white paper, 'Our Health, Our Care, Our Say: a Direction for Community Services', (2006), had set out our challenge, 'to increase EPP course capacity from 12,000 course places a year to 100,000 by 2012', (p112) through the establishment of a CIC that would become a national provider of self-management courses in England. Not only did the white paper commit to an increased course capacity but also that EPP would 'diversify and respond better to the needs of its participants. Courses will be designed to meet people's different needs, including those in marginalized groups, provide the opportunity to develop new courses, make its products available in new markets, and develop new partnerships with all stakeholders involved in self care' (p112/113).

Self-management has been available in England since the early 1990s and the generic Chronic Disease Self Management Course (CDSMC)[1] was introduced in 1998, as the Expert Patients Programme (EPP). It was managed by the DH and piloted across the English NHS from 2002 to 2004. Having been successfully piloted, the NHS EPP was rolled out across England through the primary care trusts (PCTs), still led by the DH, with day-to-day management from an NHS operational management team. During this time, the NHS EPP was run through teams based within the (then) 28 strategic health authorities (SHAs). During the pilot phase, 1,300 courses were delivered to over 17,000 people.

The 2005 Labour Party Manifesto[2] (p64) had pledged to treble investment in the EPP and this had been followed by the 2006 White Paper[1]. The DH saw this as an opportunity to expand the work already undertaken across England around self care and self-management and for EPP to have a protected financial future. The changes in PCTs around practice-based commissioning at the time meant that the current funding arrangements for the NHS EPP would not have been sustainable in the new climate. As pledged, investment in EPP was increased and the DH funded the establishment of a Community Interest Company (CIC). Once established, it was agreed that EPP–CIC would become self-funding as health and social care organizations commissioned its courses.

This was a bold experimental move for the DH and demonstrated a new way of working. The EPP was one of the first national NHS programmes to be established as a CIC, falling against a backdrop of major changes in the health service with the reorganization of SHAs in July 2006 and encouragement of PCTs to commission courses rather than provide them directly. In fact, it was a creative and interesting move for the Government as a whole. The idea of putting public funds into a company with clear goals, but relative freedom as to their achievement represented a completely different enabling philosophy to service development. The CIC structure was itself a new form of legal entity, being a not-for-profit company with social objectives. Critically a CIC has an 'asset lock'; meaning that funds put into the company, as well as any surpluses made, can only be used for reinvestment in the company's aims.

On 1 April 2007, EPP–CIC went live with its own Board of Directors chaired by Stephen Jacobs OBE. The company's purpose was defined as to: *establish the principle of individual self-management and self care as a recognised public health measure, deliverable in a cost effective and sustained way.* In line with a patient-led NHS, EPP–CIC wants self-management courses to be available to everyone living with an LTC in England, currently estimated at over 15 million people[3], and predicted to increase by 1 million every decade.

The challenge was set, with just over £16 million from the DH to establish ourselves in the market place. In 2007, we were still very much an organization working in the same way as before under the DH's governance. Now, we had to deliver a commercial product within a largely public sector commissioning environment, entailing changing the mind set, culture and skill base of the workforce. There was no corporate, financial, HR, or IT infrastructure except for an intranet system previously regulated by the DH central communications team. Our first big task was to restructure the organization. Inevitably it was a difficult time as we created a business model that would have the resources and capacity to deliver the Government's commitment while keeping the values and beliefs that had made the original programme successful. The structure required a whole new work culture for staff that created both challenges and opportunities for everyone. It also meant a different set of accountabilities, enabling clear goals and responsibilities to be embedded for everyone. The previous twin Managing Director structure was replaced by myself, as Chief Executive, with the support of an executive director team. Jean Thompson MBE retired, having done so much to establish the UK self care agenda, and achieving many of her original objectives. Her partnering managing director, Jim Phillips, stayed as part of the new executive director structure and continues to make valuable leadership contributions to the development of products and the quality of our delivery.

The 23 regional offices were restructured into 5 regions and the principles of clear goals and stronger local accountability ensued. A regional manager, business development manager, administrative support, and trainers were appointed in each region, the staff from the previous NHS programme filling the majority of these positions.

More autonomy was given to the regions with clear guidance around building local 'capacity' and the marketplace for self care at community level by developing stronger relationships within them. The regional business development managers are working with PCTs and SHAs to include self care in their local delivery plans. Local 'capacity' is developed as more people attend courses and then take up the option to become tutors themselves. An aggressive programme of tutor development became necessary.

As the public knowledge of the availability of self care training is low, it remains a challenge to improve the awareness of self care and its benefits. This not only has to be achieved at a regional level but clear key messages are also needed centrally requiring continuous refinement. Communication is an essential part of our new business plan and like the other parts of the business we need to get it right. We now have a central communications team of four led by a marketing and communications manager and a marketing lead in each regional team. We are continually exploring new ways to promote EPP–CIC and self care. In 2009, for the first time, we were one of four main sponsors at a major LTCs' event. We were pleased to be well received by the audience, and it has opened up new areas of work for us.

Although the investment from the DH was a substantial amount, we had to deploy it carefully. If we had only used it to cover course delivery costs, the fund would have been quickly exhausted without making significant inroads into the DH targets. Creation of a viable business was risky if it could only be sustained by *course delivery*, we needed to become a *centre of expertise on self care*. Our long-term future depended on successfully developing a larger market, with many more providers than ourselves. Our role would be that of a catalyst, using funding to 'pump prime' where appropriate, ensuring new products, quality standards, and delivery networks were all optimal for the new market growth.

Over the last few years, self-management and self care have become central to the Government's vision for the NHS. There has been a strong push to put the patient and their family at the centre of their own healthcare, giving them more say and control. Lord Darzi's review[4] of the NHS (2008) reflects a shift from a curative to a preventative approach, emphasizing the need to educate people about lifestyle choices and their potential impact on health.

This shift has also forced us to look at the products we have on offer. Evaluation[5] of the generic CDSMP showed that, while the personal benefits of attending a course were demonstrated, there was not always a clear reduction of health service utilization. This was no surprise as Stanford University had never made any such claims for the course, but it did make us review the services we offer and their marketing.

One way of addressing some of the issues raised in the evaluation (see Chapter 12) is our programme developed with the Health Foundation to provide a whole system approach to self-management under the Co-Creating Health initiative (see Chapter 13). We have written, and are delivering the training for four self-management disease-specific courses for people living with diabetes, chronic obstructive pulmonary disease (COPD), depression, and musculo-skeletal pain. These courses are being run in 8 sites across England. The Co-creating Health initiative not only delivers self-management programmes to patients but also works with health professionals, giving them the opportunity to learn the same set of skills to support their patients in self-managing their condition. The aim is to help health care organizations create new models of health care that embed self-management within mainstream services.

In another whole systems approach to self-management, EPP–CIC has taken over the NHS Working in Partnership Programme's (WiPP) suite of self care resources including the Self Care Connect website (www.selfcareconnect.co.uk). Within this are two self care training courses: 'Self Care for You' and 'Self Care for Primary Care', providing skills and advice to help people engage in self care to improve their lifestyle and develop positive health behaviours. These are part of the larger WiPP targeted at the general patient population. Through these two programmes, we have recognized that the facilitated workshop process at the heart of self-management tuition could be adapted to address some of the issues of biomedical progression and health service utilization that had been critically evaluated. For example, providing more time and focus on self-medication does improve patient expertise in areas that can help to reduce the progression of many conditions. The training developed as a result of this has been well received, and in June 2007 we won an Ask About Medicines Award for Excellence (under the category 'excellence in providing medicines information to medicine users and the public'). Since the establishment of EPP–CIC in 2007, we have changed and adapted our portfolio of products, targeting people living with an LTC and promoting self care and healthy well-being to everyone.

A number of courses have been developed to meet different needs including:

- Recovery from substance and alcohol misuse (SAM)
- Living with or in recovery from a mental health condition (New Beginnings)
- Adults caring for someone with a LTC or disability (Looking after Me)
- Parents or carers of children with long-term or life-limiting conditions (Supporting Parents Programme)
- A Persistent Pain Programme
- People with learning difficulties
- Health and social care practitioners needing to increase their awareness of self-management (Wise Up)
- A prison course
- People with LTCs who want to return to work (Forward Steps)

A course for people with learning disabilities will be available from 2009.

It is becoming apparent that many people attending self-management courses are already reasonably health conscious having actively sought ways to help themselves manage their condition. We have therefore recognized the need to target 'harder to reach' groups, such as those with an LTC who are unaware that there are resources available to them other than the prescribed medicines. A major area of our work has been to focus on reaching minority groups and making our courses more accessible. The CDSMP is now available in nine languages and bilingual trainers deliver this and the Looking After Me course across England.

The teams have worked hard to ensure the accessibility of our courses to our target audiences. This can mean changing the times of the courses to fit in with prayer times, caring responsibilities or just ensuring the courses are run in familiar places such as local community centres. At the beginning of 2009, the East Lancashire PCTs EPP team were awarded the two Excellence in Practice awards; 'Tackling Health Inequalities' and 'Championing Diversity'. Both recognized outreach to different minority groups in their local area and had featured specialist courses developed by EPP–CIC.

EPP–CIC now has a license to deliver the online version of the CDSMC to people who are housebound, live in rural areas or just do not like group settings. The NHS EPP successfully piloted this, courses being available nationally from May 2009 (see Ian McNeil's item in Chapter 6).

In response to a request from the DH for a self-management course for young people, a series of workshops were developed for people between 12 and 18 years old called Staying Positive (see Kathy Hawley's item in Chapter 4). It is during this period that responsibility for management of their condition often transfers from parent to the young person. The workshops not only aid awareness and management of their condition but it also assists in challenging any erroneous beliefs that may have developed. They were designed through direct consultation with young people and are run by trained young facilitators who also have experience of living with an LTC. We needed a different format to the standard CDSMC to ensure its appeal to the target audience. The workshops enable young people to share experiences, learn and practice new skills, and gain support from their peers. In November 2008, Staying Positive won the Guardian Public Services Award in the category of 'Service delivery for LTCs'. Short-listed from 850 entries, it was a fantastic achievement.

We are also investing time and resources to support people on Incapacity Benefit get back into work. As partners in the Department of Work and Pensions' 'Pathways to Work' initiative, we have secured contracts to deliver condition management training, involving individual case management and demonstrating many flexible ways that the thinking behind self-management techniques can be adapted.

In line with our corporate aim of making courses as accessible as possible for everyone, EPP–CIC is the lead administrative organization delivering a 3-year DH programme for adult, unpaid carers – Caring with Confidence. as part of the Government's New Deal for Carers and the National Carers Strategy: born, like EPP–CIC, out of the White Paper 'Our Health, Our Care, Our Say'[1]. EPP–CIC submitted a joint bid with four other organizations – Carers UK, Crossroads Caring for Carers, Partners UK, and The Princess Royal Trust for Carers. Caring with Confidence not only aims to improve the health and well-being of the carer but also the person they care for. By focussing the programme on building carers' strengths, providing them with useful information, ideas and tips, and enabling them to share their experiences with others in similar circumstances they are supported to make positive differences to their own life and that of the person they care for.

We have positioned ourselves as a leader in opening up new work for people with LTCs. Our volunteers play an integral role in the delivery of our services, indeed any course participants can sign up for training as a volunteer tutor.

For some, this can be a route back to work, but at the same time we are committed to supporting those for whom this is not an option. Each region had built up a bank of volunteer tutors whose role has been addressed within the organization. A competency framework for tutors has been devised, and by the end of 2009 we shall be introducing formal tutor accreditation in recognition that participants benefit most from well-delivered enjoyable courses. Some tutors can now be paid for their services. The aim is to increase the tutor base to 5,000 through partnership working with other voluntary sector organizations and local communities.

In the 2 years since its establishment, EPP–CIC has made great progress turning the NHS programme into a business model that, to date, is on track to meet its objective of sustainability by 2012. In our first year, as a company, we did four times as much business as had been done in similar periods previously and in 2008/2009 we did twice as much again.

To date, over 40,000 people have attended an EPP course and 1,600 have been trained as tutors. It is clear that with such a large rapidly growing group there is not only work still to be done to achieve the government's commitment to increase this to 100,000 course places a year, but we need to ensure these places are accessible to everyone who needs them. I think we are working well to achieve this, and one of our strengths has been to change and diversify according to the ever changing market and the needs of our target audience. EPP–CIC has been, and will always be, about making self-management and self care a recognized public health measure.

Endnotes

1 Chronic Disease Self Management Course – originated from Stanford University, California and created by Professor Kate Lorig.

2 The 2005 Labour Party Manifesto.

3 Department of Health www.dh.gov.uk.

4 'High Quality Care for All – NHS Next Stage Review Final Report', Department of Health, June 08.

5 Cost effectiveness of the EPP for patients with chronic conditions. G Richardson, A Kennedy, D Reeves, et al. (2008) *Journal of Epidemiology and Community Health* **62**: 361–7.

Chapter 13

Co-Creating Health: Transforming health care systems

Natalie Grazin in conversation
with Roy Jones

Co-Creating Health is a 3-year quality improvement initiative run by The Health Foundation in 8 health economies across the UK. Its aim is to test and demonstrate the feasibility of putting self-management support at the heart of mainstream health care. Moving away from stand-alone self-management courses for patients, Co-Creating Health's goal is that self-management support will be embedded throughout the health care system and be recognized as a core component of clinically excellent NHS care for people with long-term conditions.

Roy Jones: So, what was the background to the establishment of Co-Creating Health?
Natalie Grazin: The Health Foundation is a charitable body which works to improve the quality of health services across the UK and beyond. In 2004, we decided that we wanted to invest in initiatives to increase the engagement of patients in achieving better health outcomes. As an organization whose work is always grounded in evidence, we began with a review of the literature, as well as the social and policy context. This quickly led us to the conclusion that self-management was where we could help to make a difference.

What struck us was that although self-management had clearly taken off in the UK, it was very much seen as beyond the responsibility of mainstream clinical services – or at best, was at their periphery. It was generally not recognized as an aspect of good clinical care. We found that although there was lots of rhetoric and good intention around self-management support, particularly in government-level policy documents, there was remarkably little 'know-how' or even experimentation at the frontline of the NHS.

The Foundation's mission is to help the UK health services to be the best they can be. So, we decided that we should aim to get into practice the substantial evidence about the ways in which health services and clinicians could help people with their self-management. We worked with researchers and practitioners from around the world to develop a programme which would tackle all the factors which currently inhibit self-management. What we came up with is unique, we think, in terms of taking a whole system approach. The Foundation's Board approved a grant of just under £5 million late in 2006 and the 3-year initiative began in 2007. Through this, we are supporting a group of ambitious health care organizations from across the UK to create new models of health care that embed self-management support within mainstream health services.

RJ: How do you see the link between voluntary sector provision of self-management support, including the Expert Patient Programme, and what The Health Foundation is doing?

NG: Our view is that the voluntary sector and Expert Patient lay-led self-management courses, as a form of self-management support, are extremely valuable and are very effective for many people. But it's not an either/or scenario – there's more than enough need to allow the testing of different models of self-management support delivery. Arguably, it would be foolish *not* to harness the NHSs vast resources to provide at least some of that support.

What's interesting about the way that self-management support has developed is how it is positioned as something people with long-term conditions 'do' almost independently of health services. When Kate Lorig spoke at an international self-management conference in Canada in 2005, her key message was that although she'd needed to get self-management off the ground by starting outside the medical establishment, that didn't mean that it should always stay that way. Her argument was that we can only successfully build people's self-management skills on a long-term and large-scale basis when we co-opt all the hundreds of thousands of health professionals who work with people with long-term conditions into the workforce of people delivering self-management support – they need to be allies, not opponents.

The other important thing that happened around that time and which shaped our programme design was the publication of the interim evaluation of the Expert Patient Programme[1]. While much of it was positive, what particularly interested us was the evidence that very weak links between the EPP and health services, particularly medical staff and other clinicians, was limiting take-up of the programme. We were also very struck by the evaluation's comments about the absence of follow-up support for people who'd completed the EPP. It seemed to us that this was exactly why we needed to transform mainstream health services, so that patients who'd learnt the language, skills and attitudes of self-management could return to a GP, a practice nurse or a consultant who knew what they were talking about and more importantly, who themselves had the skills to help that person with their self-management.

But there's also a final argument for positioning self-management support within health services, as opposed to outside them. Research shows that most people still have enormous respect for what their clinicians tell them; doctors in particular have enormous credibility and authority with patients. So, it's vitally important to secure the engagement of health professionals in encouraging patients to learn about self-management. The EPP evaluation revealed how damaging it can be when health professionals are distrustful of self-management; we wanted to turn that on its head.

RJ: Which means that the self-management support is a continuous intervention and not a one-off?
NG: Exactly. It's the difference between seeing the classic 6-week course as if it were a one-off 'dose', rather than part of ongoing excellent clinical care. Our vision is that we reach a stage where self-management support is a core expectation of clinicians, rather than an add-on that only some clinicians deliver, or something which is delivered outside the health system.

One of the difficulties in doing this is finding the right language to ensure that people understand what we mean. The most important example is ensuring that clinicians recognise that what patients do is 'self-management' and what they can provide is 'self-management support'. In Co-Creating Health, we've used a version of Tom Bodenheimer's definition of self-management support (adapted into the UK terminology), which we find extremely helpful:

'*Self-management support is the assistance that caregivers give to people with long-term conditions in order to encourage daily decisions that improve health-related behaviours and clinical outcomes. It can be viewed in two ways:*

◆ *A portfolio of tools and techniques that help patients choose healthy behaviours*

◆ *A fundamental transformation of the patient–caregiver relationship into a collaborative partnership*'[2]

This two-part definition sums up very well what Co-Creating Health is about: on the one hand, we're re-organizing health care around a very specific and practical set of tools and techniques that are applicable in any health care context; and we're also working at a more fundamental level to transform the relationships between patients and health professionals.

RJ: How did you decide where your demonstration sites would be?
NG: We used a competitive process to select the Co-Creating Health sites, based on a range of demanding criteria including the excellence of the existing service; a style of work that had the potential to develop into true collaboration with patients; strong clinical leadership; and critically, senior organizational support. Eight superb teams (listed in Appendix 1) were finally chosen,

spanning four long-term conditions: COPD, depression, diabetes, and musculoskeletal pain.

We wanted a range of long-term conditions within the initiative so that we could generate strong evidence about what works. Our choice of which long-term conditions to include was influenced by a very interesting piece of original research undertaken for us by the Picker Institute in 2005; this used Judith Hibbard's Patient Activation Measure to assess the self-efficacy of people living with a variety of long-term conditions and it revealed that the conditions that are consistently associated with lower self-management ability are depression, chronic pain, bladder, bowel, and gastric conditions[3]. So, in order to ensure that our work was designed to support even those starting with the lowest levels of self-efficacy, we wanted to include at least two of these conditions within our initiative – hence the inclusion of chronic pain and depression alongside COPD and diabetes.

RJ: Could you explain what 'the three enablers' are within Co-Creating Health and why they're important?
NG: The enablers are the 3-key processes that facilitate effective self-management support within a clinical relationship. They effectively re-structure interactions between patients and clinicians so that they change from the traditional dynamic to one of a collaborative interaction. Tom Bodenheimer has a great description of the differences between these two types of relationship, and in Co-Creating Health we've used an adapted version of his model as follows[4]:

Traditional interactions	Collaborative interactions
Information is given and skills taught based on the clinician's agenda	Patient and clinician share their agendas and collaboratively decide what information is needed and which skills should be taught
The clinician's starting point is that knowledge creates behaviour change	The clinician's starting point is that the patient's confidence in their ability to change ('self-efficacy'), together with knowledge, creates behaviour change
The patient believes it is the clinician's role to improve health	The patient believes that they have an active role to play in changing their own behaviours to improve their own health
Goals are set by the clinician and success is measured by compliance with them	The patient is supported by the clinician in defining their own goals. Success is measured by an ability to attain those goals
Decisions are made by the clinician, possibly informed by their understanding of the patient's preferences	Decisions are explicitly made as a patient–clinician partnership

Data from Bodenheimer 2005

The three 'enablers' are the structured processes which ensure that interactions are collaborative and empowering. They'll be very familiar with anyone who's facilitated or participated in a self-management programme because there's a great similarity with the action planning process at the core of the Stanford course and many other self-management programmes: the aim overall is to tap into people's existing wishes and hopes and start a process of building their confidence and belief in their capacity to affect their health and reduce their dependence on the clinician. In Co-Creating Health, we're bringing that process into the clinician–patient dynamic and engaging the support of the clinical team to help the patient with setting and achieving their goals.

The first enabler is agenda setting. This requires that patients and clinicians explicitly and jointly agree the aims of each meeting. This helps to establish the patient's own motivations and interests in order that the clinician can work with them to improve the relevance of the advice given and ensure that the goals chosen clearly relate to the patient's concerns, desires, and priorities. The Co-Creating Health sites are using a wide variety of tools to help patients to identify and prioritise their agenda; many of these are very simple prompts which patients receive along with their appointment letter or just before the appointment and then bring into the consultation with them. Bubble sheets are a very popular way of giving this prompt (Fig. 13.1):

Agenda-setting at the start of any meeting between clinician and patient transforms the dynamic between them. If you think about any other aspect of your life, for example, meeting your bank manager, you would expect to have a part in agreeing the objectives for your meeting!

The next enabler is goal setting. This step supports patients to set short-term goals which will help them to build their self-efficacy. The goals may or may not be clinical in nature, but they should be of real importance to the patient. The clinicians are taught to support the patient to develop a realistic action plan around their goal, much as the patient would have done each week during a self-management course.

The last enabler is goal follow-up. Essentially, this is a proactive contact from the health care team to support patients with achieving the goals they've set. Goal follow-up is probably the most difficult enabler to introduce effectively, because it requires system change and goes beyond changing the process of a single consultation. While it might be a GP, practice nurse, physiotherapist or a consultant, or who agrees the goal with a patient, it's quite possibly someone else within the team who contacts them to say, 'Hi, it's a few days since you set your goal, I hope you're feeling good about it, how's it going?'. That needs to happen reliably as a property of the system: the follow-up might be done by a receptionist well trained in motivational interviewing, by a practice nurse, or

My Diabetes Plan

How are you doing with your diabetes?

☐ Excellent   ☐ Good   ☐ Not Good   ☐ Not sure

I am doing well with:

☐ Exercising

☐ Eating better foods

☐ Taking my medicine

☐ Checking my blood sugar

☐ Managing my weight

☐ Reducing my salt intake

☐ Cutting down on smoking

☐ Checking my feet

☐ Drinking less alcohol

☐ Other

I want to do better with:

☐ Exercising

☐ Eating better foods

☐ Taking my medicine

☐ Checking my blood sugar

☐ Managing my weight

☐ Reducing my salt intake

☐ Setting a quit smoking date

☐ Checking my feet

☐ Drinking less alcohol

☐ Other

To improve my health, I will work on one of my chosen activities.

This is what I am going to do: _____

How much: _____

When: _____

How often: _____

How important is this activity to me? (circle a number)
Not   1   2   3   4   5   6   7   8   9   10   Very

How confident am I that I will be able to do this activity? (circle a number)
Not   1   2   3   4   5   6   7   8   9   10   Very

Fig. 13.1 Sample agenda-setting bubble sheet (as used by the Co-Creating Health team in NHS Haringay, NHS Islington, and the Whittington Hospital NHS Trust).

With kind permission of Natalie Grazin, Co-Creating Health team, NHS Haringay, NHS Islington, and the Whittington Hospital NHS Trust indeed by a telephone-based qualified nurse or a health coach who supports the patients from across many clinics or practices. Implementing this enabler has been hard; the default is still to see follow-up as part of a next or 'follow-up' appointment, which may be too late to be effective in terms of reinforcing goal motivation. In order for this enabler to be delivered efficiently and cost-effectively, a different system and possibly even a different workforce may be needed, which is why this is the hardest enabler to implement.

RJ: So, how does Co-Creating Health work in practice? What's actually happening within each site to bring about these changes?
NG: Each site participating in Co-Creating Health receives an integrated package of support for a period of three years, delivered on-site and at national meetings by a team of experts. Over time, the capability and capacity of the site to be self-sustaining in further rolling out this approach is built up through a train-the-trainer approach. The activities on each site include:

- An **Advanced Development Programme for Clinicians** – this supports clinicians to develop the skills required to support and motivate their patients to take an active role in their own health
- A **Self-Management Programme for people with long-term conditions** – this supports patients to develop the knowledge and skills they require in order to manage their long-term condition and work in effective partnership with their clinicians
- A **Service Improvement Programme** – this supports patients and health care professionals, working together, to identify and implement new approaches to health service delivery which enable patients to take a more active role in their own health

In addition, we hold a 9-monthly 'National Forum' where around 100 people from across all the demonstration sites, including clinicians and patients, come together to learn from each other and to hear from the UK and international experts. The whole initiative is being independently and externally evaluated by Coventry University (see Chapter 14).

RJ: How does Co-Creating Health encourage clinicians to change their approach and to build their self-management support skills?
NG: The Advanced Development Programme for clinicians is designed to strengthen the skills and knowledge health professionals need to provide self-management support, focusing particularly on the 'three enablers'. The 9-month programme consists of three half-day workshops co-facilitated by a local health professional and a local patient, web-based learning; and ongoing

action learning sets designed to support participants with fully implementing the skills they've learnt on the course. The workshops for clinicians use active learning methods such as role-play and video. They give clinicians a safe environment to learn, test, and refine new approaches to their consultation, with trained actors playing patients. They can practice and 'rewind' conversations with the actors over and over again until they find a form of words that works for them.

It's extraordinary to observe how difficult it can be for many clinicians to change their consultation practice. Observing the workshops, you see many clinicians who understand the theory and buy into what they're learning – indeed, they are often very excited by the approach. But when they come to actually try it out, it's hard – simply because their consultation pattern and language has become deeply ingrained and changing any behaviour that's become habitual is such a challenge.

The other barrier for many clinicians is their sense of their responsibility to provide optimum care for their patients, including their responsibility to make sure that the patient has heard the necessary advice. So, it's important that clinicians find an approach which feels comfortable and safe in terms of balancing risk and professional responsibility with sufficiently open collaboration around goal-setting. It's all too easy to characterize clinicians and doctors particularly, as behaving in a paternalistic way for negative reasons, but for many, they are genuinely motivated by responsibility as well as a fear of providing negligent care. We think that it's important to ensure that clinicians are aware of the guidelines from the GMC and the Royal Colleges which do support shared decision-making and collaborative consultation processes, as long as they're well-recorded, evidence-based and include a sensible approach to risk management. So, issues about the culture of health care, responsibility, and risk are major lessons that have come up for us and reflect the wider context in which we're operating.

RJ: I'm interested by the co-facilitation of the clincians' Advanced Development Programme by a local clinician and a local patient. What is the logic for doing this?
NG: Traditionally, patients' involvement in clinician training has been as 'exhibits' – passive clinical material on which clinicians can develop their skills. Until recently, their experience and perspective has been almost entirely untapped as a source of teaching. In designing Co-Creating Health, we felt that it was key that this social modelling was part of the training experience; we want the clinicians participating in the programme to work with their patients in a partnership mode – what better way to encourage this than to model it

through the way the course is delivered? It gives an example to the participants of partnership working in practice. This has however been one of the hardest aspects of Co-Creating Health to implement consistently across the 8 sites. Patients are not fully empowered to co-deliver the course in every site yet – the mental health sites, for example, are able to adopt the model much more effectively than most other sites. But I'm confident that it will eventually happen in all sites – it's important and powerful when it works well.

RJ: *Finally, what would you say have been the key pieces of learning so far from Co-Creating Health?*
NG: Firstly, the importance of context. NHS organizations that have a genuine corporate commitment to collaboration with patients seem to be able to succeed better than others. It makes a great difference when Boards, Chief Executives, and clinical leaders see this agenda as a genuine organisational priority, rather than as an 'add on'.

Secondly, we've learnt a lot about clinicians' engagement in self-management support. Much of this work involves addressing deeply held personal beliefs and long-established practices. These attitudes and beliefs are set early in their training and reinforced as clinicians go along. We have to be mindful of this, seek to understand it and support clinicians to work through those beliefs both intellectually and emotionally. We've also learnt that clinician champions are vital for persuading other clinicians to come on board; the clinical leads in each of our 8 sites play a central and irreplaceable role in influencing other clinicians to become involved in Co-Creating Health.

Thirdly, the challenge of measuring the effectiveness of this work is a big and ongoing issue. Accounts from patients of how self-management has changed their lives emerged fairly quickly and these are often moving and compelling. More unusually, we've also got narratives from clinicians outlining the profound effects that this work has had on their clinical practice, their attitudes, and their satisfaction with their own roles. What's harder for us to demonstrate at this mid-term point is the sort of hard outcomes data that would constitute the evidence that some audiences such as commissioners may want – but we hope that this will happen as the initiative continues and as the external evaluation completes its work.

Finally, the most important thing we've learnt is the importance of holding firm to our own 'whole system' approach. The greatest success stories are from those settings where all three parts of the initiative – work with clinicians, patients, and service improvement – are all happening. Each reinforces the other and no one part of the initiative alone could have the effectiveness that the three are having together.

Acknowledgement

Thanks to colleagues within The Health Foundation; to the Co-Creating Health National Support Team and Programme Office; and most of all, to the teams in the eight Co-Creating Health sites.

Appendix – Co-Creating Health sites

COPD

- NHS Ayrshire and Arran
- Cambridge University Hospitals NHS Foundation Trust, Cambridgeshire Primary Care Trust

Diabetes

- Guy's & St. Thomas' NHS Foundation Trust, Southwark Health, and Social Care
- Whittington NHS Hospital Trust, Islington PCT, Haringey PCT

Depression

- South West London & St. George's Mental Health NHS Trust, Wandsworth Teaching PCT
- Devon Partnership Trust, Torbay Care Trust

Musculoskeletal pain

- Calderdale and Huddersfield NHS Foundation Trust, Calderdale PCT, Kirklees PCT
- North Bristol NHS Trust, Bristol Primary Care Trust

Endnotes

1 Kennedy A, Gately C, Rogers A. *Process Evaluation of the EPP – Report II: Examination of the implementation of the Expert Patients Programme within the structures and locality contexts of the NHS in England.* University of Manchester, National Primary Care Research and Development Centre, 2005.

2 Bodenheimer T., MacGregor K., Sharifi C., *Helping Patients Manage Their Chronic Conditions,* California Health Foundation, 2005.

3 Ellins J., Coulter A., *How Engaged are People in their Healthcare?* The Health Foundation, 2005.

4 Bodenheimer T et al., ibid.

Chapter 14

Three bodies of the UK research

The 3 writers in this chapter make very different contributions. Julie Barlow has researched/evaluated many self-management projects since the outset in 1993. The lead in many studies, she has contributed to many others. Anne Kennedy led the trial team which conducted a national evaluation of the EPP and together with Anne Rogers, writes for the team at the National Primary Care R&D Centre in Manchester where several studies connected to the trial were run. This is the largest multi-centred study to date. Louise Wallace is the other professor with Julie Barlow in the Applied Research Department at Coventry. Her team is conducting the research and evaluation programme for the Health Foundation's Co-Creating Health programme.

Coventry University

Julie Barlow

This section presents a summary of our studies of the Stanford arthritis and chronic disease courses conducted by the team at Coventry University over a period of 16 years and includes the key learning points derived from conducting these studies.

Arthritis Self-Management Programme (ASMP)

Arthritis Care introduced this course in the early 1990s and it has been evaluated in a range of delivery settings and modes of recruitment. The first evaluation in the UK was focused on older people with arthritis (i.e. over 55 years) using a pre-post test design. Results after 4 months demonstrated significant improvements in arthritis self-efficacy, generalized self-efficacy, depression, positive affect, cognitive symptom management, communication with doctors, pain, exercise, relaxation, and visits to primary care practitioners. We learned that the benefits of a course may be wide-ranging at least among this group. A small, statistically significant improvement in generalized self-efficacy suggested it influenced perceived ability to cope with the demands faced everyday by older people with arthritis. Hence, we learned that improvements are not limited to managing arthritis per se but may generalize to other areas of life. We learned that despite the group format that provided the opportunity to meet with similar others and share of experiences, there was no change in satisfaction with social support at 4-month follow-up. Perhaps, any change in social support is short-lived unless the participants establish their own supportive network. This problem of termination of support at the end of an intervention is not specific to the ASMP, but inherent in many short courses.

Since then, we have conducted a series of evaluations covering a range of populations and delivery settings in the UK. In a randomized, controlled trial (RCT) we had a sample of 544 participants (84% female) with a mean age of 58 years, mean disease duration of 11 years. Fifty-two percent had osteoarthritis (OA), 35% had rheumatoid arthritis (RA), and 13% had other types of arthritis, confirmed by their GPs. Analysis revealed that at 4-month follow-up, the course had a significant effect on arthritis self-efficacy, use of self-management behaviours and depressed mood. This range, noted earlier, was largely confirmed using the more rigorous design of an RCT. The effect sizes tend to be moderate for self-efficacy and small for other outcome variables (e.g. 43 for arthritis self-efficacy and 27 for communication with physicians and depressed mood). However, not only were improvements maintained but significant decreases in pain and visits to GPs were evident in the 12-month follow-up. We learned that apart from a small improvement in physical functioning at 12-months among the intervention group with OA, results were independent of type of arthritis. Finally, we learned that the UK attracts more people with RA into the course than typically reported in US studies (i.e. approximately 40 versus 14%). This makes a difference to the level of physical functioning across the sample, suggesting greater impairment in UK samples.

Results of a nested qualitative study based on interviews with intervention group participants showed perceived increased confidence (self-efficacy), and felt they have the 'tools' and motivation to make changes. Within the group setting of course delivery, participants share information, compare themselves with similar others (social comparisons), experience role modelling, and feel they have found an appropriate peer group helping to reduce their sense of isolation. Thus, the qualitative findings shed some light on 'how' participants change during the ASMP.

An 8-year follow-up of the original intervention group ($n = 125$) in 2000, suggests that may be maintained in the longer term, (published, 2008). The exception was the physical functioning score, that was stable from baseline to 4-months (as expected), but increased at 8-years indicating a decline. We learned that despite a decline in physical functioning, course participants' maintained self-efficacy, psychological well-being, and use of self-management techniques. Interviews were conducted with a sub-sample of 10 participants (5 with low self-efficacy and 5 with high self-efficacy). Despite the gap of 8 years, participants easily recalled their experience of course attendance. This has been linked to emotionally salient events (Pashler, 2002) suggesting that for some, ASMP attendance was a significant event. This was evident when some participants talked about not having had a future before the ASMP. The main difference between high- and low self-efficacy interviewees concerned pre-course expectations: low self-efficacy participants expressed disappointment that the course was not a medical treatment or instant cure. The latter is consistent with wishful thinking (itself a type of passive, emotion-focused coping) and accords with difficulty accepting the condition and its psychosocial consequences. From this follow-up study, we learned there may be a need to address illness representations before some participants are able to fully engage with the ASMP and that some people need more psychological support than can be provided in a short, lay-led intervention.

The Coventry team was involved in a RCT lead by Buszewicz and colleagues. This trial focused on patients with OA aged 50+ ($n = 812$) recruited through 74 general practices across the UK (1). The intervention group received the ASMP and an education booklet, whereas the control group received just the booklet. At 12-month follow-up, there was significant impact from the ASMP in terms of improvement in anxiety and arthritis self-efficacy for pain and other symptoms. A significant difference in depression was noted at 4-month follow-up, but was not evident at 12-months. There was no difference in GP visits at 12 months. Approximately, 30% of the intervention group failed to attend any of the course sessions. Telephone interviews revealed that the main reasons for non-attendance were the timing of the course or difficulties associated with accessing the venue. There was no impact on health care usage contrasting with the results of the US studies of the ASMP (Lorig & Holman, 1993), where large reductions in visits to physicians are reported. When the ASMP was first introduced here, there was debate about the potential for increasing demand on health services following course attendance. However, studies consistently show that there is little impact on health care utilization. This finding may work against the commissioning of courses where the sole intention is to reduce health care costs.

Chronic Disease Self-management Course (CDSMC)

ASMP paved the way for the development and implementation of the generic Chronic Disease Self-Management Course (CDSMC). The Long-Term Medical

Conditions Alliance (now National Voice) delivered it in 2000 within the Living with Long-term Illness (LILL) project. Participants' range of long-term health conditions included arthritis, endometriosis, depression, diabetes, myalgic encephalomyelitis, osteoporosis, and polio. Improvements identified at 4-month follow-up (published 2003), included increased self-efficacy, decreased fatigue, depressed moods, and health distress. These were maintained at 12-months and participants reported sustained use of self-management skills (e.g. cognitive symptom management, communication skills). Furthermore, participants used this course for sharing experiences and used goal setting to help make changes. In essence, the generic course provided participants with the confidence to select the self-management techniques (or tools) that met their specific needs and helped them to develop the necessary competencies (published 2005). We learned that the CDSMC had the potential to provide similar benefits to the ASMP across a range of different conditions. We have since examined the effectiveness of the CDSMC in two RCTs focusing on specific target groups.

We examined the effectiveness of the CDSMC for Myocardial Infarction (MI) patients in a RCT ($n = 192$, mean age 65.9 years and a median duration of 1 year since their first MI) (published 2009). All participants had completed Cardiac Rehabilitation within the previous 2 years. This CDSMC was run exclusively for MI patients and was delivered by two lay tutors who had had heart attacks. There were no statistically significant differences between the intervention and control groups although a pattern of small improvements among the intervention group on self-efficacy, anxiety, depression, and cognitive symptom management was observed. This sample was mainly men (72%) and the duration since their first MIs was relatively short (i.e. median of 1 year) contrasting with most other studies of lay-led self-management, where the majority of participants are women and mean disease duration tends to be 10 years plus. Participants in this study were relatively high in self-efficacy and self-management competencies as may be expected among MI patients who have recently completed cardiac rehabilitation. We learned from interviews that intervention group participants perceived an overlap between the CDSMC and cardiac rehabilitation around diet and exercise. However, they viewed cardiac rehabilitation as being more about instruction, whereas CDSMC was more about discussion, mutual support, and goal setting. Interestingly, we learned that whereas women valued the emotional support provided within the CDSMC, men preferred the informational support: there are few additional benefits for this target group. However, the CDSMC may have a valuable role to play in providing the additional support needed by the most vulnerable patients, such as those who are anxious or lacking in confidence or motivation to carry out important treatment recommendations such as exercise.

Our second RCT of the CDSMC focused on people with Multiple Sclerosis (MS), but was open to anyone with a long-term health condition. Thus, participants with MS learned alongside participants with conditions such as asthma, diabetes, or heart disease (published, 2009). Results showed that at 4-months, the course was effective in terms of self-efficacy and depression although effect sizes were small but improvements were maintained at 12-months. The study included a design to examine the characteristics of people with MS who expressed an interest and received information but did not attend. This group of 'informed non-attenders' was invited to take part in a Comparison Group. These 'informed non-attenders' had longer disease duration, were less anxious, and at baseline experienced less fatigue and psychological impact. A nested qualitative study based on interviews (published, 2009) revealed that MS participants compared themselves to participants with similar symptoms, but not necessarily the same diagnosis and drew inspiration and hope from those who were coping well. From this, we learned that the use of social comparisons across and within diagnostic groupings can be beneficial, suggesting that generic self-management interventions do not compromise opportunities for making relevant informative comparisons. Participants learned that achieving small, realistic goals enhanced self-efficacy and led to feelings of empowerment and positive outlook. Again, competencies were generalized to other situations not directly connected to MS, such as parenting, social activities, and work. Equally, as in studies of the ASMP, we learned that, although participants felt more in control of their MS, many reported that they had not learned any new information or skills; rather in the CDSMC they had reinforced and honed existing competencies. Nonetheless, participants had learned to manage illness around their lives as opposed to managing their lives around their illness. From this study, we learned that people who *choose not* to enroll may be those who are coping well. Equally, many people with experience of living with long-term health conditions who developed repertoires of coping skills may yet require a course that focuses on specific issues such as working or parenting with a long-term health condition.

Attention turned to the CDSMC, when adopted as the foundation of the DoHs Expert Patient Programme (EPP), and how the course could be implemented in different settings. We conducted a longitudinal, interview-based study focusing on delivery of the EPP inside the NHS (published, 2007). As with our other studies (see 2002), participating NHS employees enjoyed being with similar others, which engendered feelings of peer belonging, acceptance, and reduced isolation. These participants valued having time to focus on their own health needs. However, they believed the EPP to be more about *living* with a long-term health condition rather than *working* with it and wanted more time spent on work connected strategies such as obtaining managerial support. Despite much publicity only 2 out of 7 managers interviewed were familiar with the EPP and there was some confusion regarding the term 'expert patient', which several managers associated with initiatives to improve standards of care. However, two managers who were aware of the EPP expressed support for staff attending the EPP or training as tutors, with the caveat that such support had to be balanced against the need to ensure that service provision was maintained not a drain on financial resources. Overall, we learned that knowledge about self-management courses cannot be assumed.

A preliminary evaluation of the Supporting Parents Programme (SPP) pilot course developed for parents of children living with a long-term health conditions was published 2008. Based on the CDSMC, the SPP aimed to empower parents to feel more able to cope with life caring for their children. The perspectives of parent participants and tutors were examined in focus groups and telephone interviews. At the end of the programme, parents reported using some of the skills learned including reflective listening, deep breathing, guided imagery, communication, and problem solving. We learned again these techniques which had been generalized to other aspects of parents' lives (e.g. work) and had been shared with their children. Although some parents felt they had not learned any new information or skills, they nonetheless perceived a commonality of emotions and practical issues, valued meeting similar others, felt less isolated, more positive, motivated, and calmer; some had found the 'real me again'. The key learning point concerned the need for continued support after the course. Parents felt that they were being cast adrift at the end of the SPP and in danger of losing the positive changes. It may be that for those who have just commenced making positive changes, long-term support is needed to maintain changes. We also discovered that lay tutors required more support and training around child protection and confidentiality; and, there is a need for a course focusing on parents of children with behavioural difficulties or ADHD. These pose specific problems for parents who felt strongly that these conditions were not amenable to change.

Lay tutors

Participants who train as course tutors develop further self-management and other competencies. We conducted several studies of tutors on both courses and published in 2001, 2003, 2004, and 2006. The studies showed that the commonest motivational factor for becoming a tutor is a desire to feel valued by helping other people. In essence, becoming a lay tutor provides the opportunity to benefit from an act of altruism. The experience of tutoring was positively reinforced by observing participants making improvements and receiving positive feedback. Lay tutors with long-term health conditions are cited as a valued aspect by course participants. This is important, given that tutors act as role models for participants. Some tutors had retired earlier than expected because of their long-term health conditions. For these, becoming course tutors resulted in a renewed sense of feeling useful and valued members of society. In a longitudinal study, where questionnaire data were collected before and after delivering the ASMP, we observed improvements in self-efficacy and psychological distress (published, 2001). However, a RCT is needed to examine this issue more rigorously. The volunteering aspect needs to be teased out to discover whether becoming lay tutor leads to better health and well-being or vice versa. Finally, we learned that the benefits of tutoring were balanced against the challenges involved.

Three main learning points to emerge from Coventry University studies of the ASMP and CDSMC (in the EPP)

Outcomes

There is increasing evidence that the impact of self-management courses resides in the psychosocial domain: there is little or no impact on health service usage in the UK studies. However, we have consistently found an improvement in positive affect. Added to this, qualitative studies suggest that participants may improve in ways that are not currently being measured. For example, tutors report transferring newly acquired skills to other areas such as advocacy groups or other community support networks. Some participants report that they are able to enrol on an educational course or seek employment. So, while many participants with long-term health conditions have already developed their own coping repertoire and fail to learn anything new from either course, most appear to enjoy the experience and gain from being reminded of techniques used in the past.

There is no lasting improvement in social support after the course and some participants feel they are being 'cast adrift'. Ways to support those who remain in need could be examined. Pre-course expectations differentiated between those low and high self-efficacy and centred on unrealistic hopes that the ASMP would provide a 'quick fix'. Such expectations were associated with lack of disease acceptance, suggesting that identifying such participants at enrolment and providing the additional support they require will be important.

Improvements may be maintained over long periods of time despite a decline in physical functioning. Further studies are needed here too.

Generalization of techniques learned

Improvement in self-efficacy is not limited to managing aspects of a long-term health conditions; there can be an increase in generalised self-efficacy for managing other aspects of life. This is perhaps not surprising given the nature of techniques such as problem solving, relaxation, and action planning. This learning point confirms that it is time to expand the range of outcomes assessed.

Mechanisms of action

The course format and process is important and provides participants with opportunities for social comparison, role modelling, inspiration and mutual exchange of coping experiences. Social comparison can be made across, as well as within, long-term health conditions. Women value the emotional aspects of a course whereas men place greater value on informational aspects. People who choose not to attend may be those who are managing better.

Conclusion

A major learning point is to remain realistic about the extent of outcomes that can be expected from a course delivered in 6 sessions by volunteer lay tutors. We know people with long-term health conditions develop innovative ways of managing their condition and applying the self-management techniques learned on these courses. Generalizing, this learning ripples out to many aspects of life.

Resources

All our published studies are listed in the Coventry University catalogue:
    The book I would recommend is Albert Bandura's *Self-Efficacy and the Exercise of Control* ISBN 0716728508.

The National Primary Care Research and Development Centre, University of Manchester

Anne Kennedy and Anne Rogers

A Researcher's view of the Expert Patients Programme

The national evaluation of the Expert Patients Programme (EPP) was carried out by a team of researchers based at the NPCR&DC at the University of Manchester. From a research viewpoint, and in a number of respects the evaluation was very successful and resulted in a number of publications and additional studies[1].

We used a range of methods for the national evaluation of the pilot phase of the EPP:

- A randomized controlled trial (RCT) to find out whether the course improved patients' outcomes and was cost-effective for the NHS
- A personal experience study to examine patients' experience of undertaking the EPP training and to compare the experience, ways of living with a long-term condition (LTC), personal self-management strategies and use of services *prior* to and *after* attending the training programme
- A process evaluation to study implementation by Primary Care Trusts (PCTs) and to find out how differing local contexts influenced the running of the programme

Other work related to the EPP

Our involvement with the national evaluation allowed us to undertake a large number of additional studies and the analysis of the data from our work related to the roll-out of the EPP has improved our understanding of the complexities of trying to engage patients and professionals with self-management. Other research related to the EPP has included:

- A survey of the volunteer tutors who facilitate the courses
- A case study of a condition specific course run in the voluntary sector (the Positive Self-Management Programme)
- A qualitative study of prisoners' perspectives of the EPP
- A qualitative study of GP and Practice nurses' views
- The case of 'living wills' training and the EPP
- A qualitative evaluation of the EPP online course
- A discrete choice experiment to determine how much patients value psychological outcomes in the context of self-management
- Conceptual work around self care support

Is the Expert Patients Programme effective?

The effectiveness of the 6-week course was measured in a randomized controlled trial that examined changes in self-efficacy (feelings of control and confidence in the management of LTCs), energy (a health outcome relevant to people with a range of LTCs) and health-related quality of life (defined in terms of health status across five dimensions: mobility, self care, usual activities, pain/discomfort, and anxiety/depression), as well as overall costs. (2) On average, the course had a marked positive impact on self-efficacy, a smaller impact on reported energy[2], and improved patients' quality of life by providing them with the equivalent of 1 extra week of perfect health per year. Although reductions in health services use were not statistically significant, (2) the cost-effectiveness analysis showed the programme was likely to be cost-effective because the reductions in service use offset the costs of providing the lay-led self care skills course. Other recent studies of variations of the Stanford Chronic Disease Self-Management Programme (CDSMC) in England support the general findings of our EPP evaluation (1, 3), although a study in an underprivileged, ethnic minority population (3) did not show the programme to be cost-effective.

The need to look beyond the delivery of self care skills training

Evaluations of the process of implementation and of the experience of patients attending the course helped to explain the trial results and highlighted the implications of running the EPP within the NHS. Several key issues emerged.

Effectiveness

Improved self-efficacy and the group experience of meeting others were valued by participants. A discrete choice exercise to determine how much participants in the trial valued self-efficacy compared with other health-related outcomes showed that participants were willing to trade substantial reductions in their health related quality of life for improvements in their self-efficacy (4). The course reinforced the value and salience of individuals' existing self care activities, but did not cause significant behaviour change. Social support from the group during the programme was also highly valued. The lay leaders were very committed to the EPP and were generally appreciated by participants, although the perceived success of the group was dependent on their facilitation skills (5). These latter aspects are the benefits of a community delivered course and would be difficult to replicate within traditional health service settings.

Self-efficacy refers to the strength of a person's belief in their capability to do a specific task or achieve a certain result (i.e. manage symptoms or engage in self-help), and is enhanced through a number of mechanisms, the most effective of which is considered to be 'performance attainment' (i.e. actual experience of the success of actions). Self-efficacy is viewed as a mediating construct for behavioural change in the EPP because changes in health status and behaviour are thought to be mediated by changes in 'self-efficacy' (6).

It is clear that self-efficacy is a desirable attribute associated with LTC manage-ment and, as an outcome, was highly valued amongst recruits of the EPP trial during its pilot phase. However, the relevance of the concept self-efficacy may be in danger of being overplayed. The emphasis placed on self-efficacy in reports of research and in the delivery of courses means that, unintentionally perhaps, it has moved from being viewed as a mediating construct to attaining the status of the most important patient outcome, bringing with it the marginalizing of other patient considerations. For example, a qualitative study found that some peoples' expectations and problems were not adequately dealt with by the course because the self care skills training programme prioritized improve-ments in self-efficacy and did not engage with patients' material and social needs (7). Moreover, the group dynamics that the EPP relies on may inadvert-ently encourage feelings of worthlessness and thus contribute to inequalities. Social comparisons, which group-based programs rely on for mediating self-efficacy, can have a negative effect if positive comparisons by individuals cannot be made. Being poor and ill brings with it the possibility of shame and insecu-rity that have the potential to be reinforced in group situations (8).

Implementation and reach

The EPP was a key policy initiative from the Department of Health that arose out of concern for the impact of LTCs on the health status of the nation along-side a need to manage demand and deal with rising costs. Expectations as to what the new policy could deliver were high and the benefits of supporting self care were certainly promoted as substantial by its advocates. Benefits identified in policy documents included: increases in life expectancy, better control over symptoms, reductions in pain, anxiety, and depression levels, improvement in quality of life with greater independence, reduction in days off work and an increase in social capital.

Health care system improvements included improved quality of consulta-tions and substantial reductions in service use.

In terms of a policy promoted as a public health initiative and against a back-ground of health policy strongly committed to tackling inequalities in health the apparent lack of patient and professional engagement with the course and the dislocation of the course from other chronic disease management being provided in the NHS proved to be a major weakness. 'Reach' is defined as the number, proportion and representativeness of individuals who participate in a given programme. Clinically and cost-effectively, the reach of the EPP has remained limited (5), and reaching more diverse and disadvantaged groups has been a challenge for CDSMP courses here and elsewhere (9). This problem might also be linked to the values that are espoused by such courses that fail to resonate with the diversity and complexity both of values and peoples' existing adaptations and perspectives on long term conditions.

In its pilot phase, the course generally attracted people who already viewed themselves as good self-managers and socio-demographic data has shown that nationally, EPP participants appeared to be better educated, live in better housing (more affluent) and are more likely to be female, than respondents to the 2003 Health Survey for England who reported at least one LTC (5). Yet, as indicated by an analysis to find out what predicts benefit from attending the EPP course (10), it is people from disadvantaged communities who may stand to benefit most from the course and if additional efforts are not made to recruit people from these communities self care support training may act to increase rather than reduce inequalities. Generic courses are hard to market if they are not targeted at a specific group of people suffering from a particular condition and are unlikely to suit everyone. Self-management initiatives need to acknowledge the diverse nature of people suffering from specific conditions who might benefit from self care support and it seems important to ensure a range of provision.

The image of an ideal Expert Patient formulated at policy level is concerned more with the type of person the patients should become, than what patients should do to maintain their health. The required type of patient is one with attributes which resonate with the responsible citizen evident in recent policy associated with New Labour welfare policies (11). There has been a proliferation of terms representing an idealized self-managing individual ('empowered', 'autonomous', 'future', 'expert', 'activated', 'wireless', 'co-producer', or 'flat pack patient'). The ideal type/notion of patient-hood demands the capacity of being confident, in control, able to monitor and manage a condition, engage with technological innovations, while at the same time allowing constraints on the demands made on services. The imposed imagery of the Expert Patient clearly lacks resonance and appeal to those it is aimed to win over. This is indicated by poor recruitment and attendance in key population groups.

Other research has highlighted problems with how individuals relate to the course content, in particular, the session on advanced care planning and living wills (12). Chronic illness is a disruptive event and people have to work to adapt to life with a LTC. The juxtaposition of educational material on healthy living with material on death and dying within the same course led to emotive, negative views that for some people, was upsetting and opened wounds. While this section was appreciated by some, it serves to demonstrate that a 'one size fits all' approach to self-management education is unlikely to be beneficial and the diverse views and experiences across age groups and ethnic minority groups regarding death and dying add to the problems of a generic approach.

The location and embedding of self care support within health service settings also requires attention. Utilization needs to be understood more broadly as part of a complex pre-existing relationship that individuals have with health care services (13). Impacts of the EPP course on health service utilization may have been limited because demand for many NHS services is, to a degree, 'supply led' (e.g. initiated by health care professionals for ongoing tests, routine monitoring, and repeat prescriptions) and also because the EPP was not designed to fit in closely with existing professional and organizational ways of working with LTCs. In theory, self-management education is linked to the ability to reduce demand for services through a process of raising the confidence and awareness of individuals to better manage their chronic condition, which in turn leads to less of a necessity to utilise health services. Even though trial results show that attending EPP courses increases self efficacy, this has so far failed to produce the promised changes in self-management. Many people do not appear to make the connection with the implicit messages transmitted via EPP that they could reduce their need for medical care by changing their behaviour. Understanding the relationship between utilization and self-management education requires moving beyond viewing outcomes in terms of increases or decreases in utilization. There is a need to view it as dynamic and part of a broader system mediated by patients' life/world experience of chronic illness and trajectories of utilisation. Services and the support provided by health professionals, and the self care that patients perform, are intrinsically linked, in that the way a person manages their condition is shaped by contact with services.

One other problem with the EPP, as it was delivered during the pilot phase, was the schism that arose between the delivery of self care skills training and the care and support provided by health professionals – particularly those working in primary care. Peer led training has its merits, most importantly that participants are able to relate to those delivering the course because of a shared history of living with a LTC. Yet, there is currently little evidence that peer-led training is superior to that delivered by professionals. We know from research that interactions with professionals are central and it maybe that the nature of relationality needs to be more of a focus rather than the technology in self care initiatives. Subjectively, people encountering self-help as an option find difficulty in limiting the professional role to that of facilitator (14). Indeed, a threat to existing positive relationships with professionals in primary care may be an unintended consequence of the lay versus professional dichotomy engendered by the promotion of peer leadership of the EPP. This is not to deny problems or issues relating to the acknowledgement of patient agendas within health professional consultations. There is evidence of a tendency of professionals to marginalize patient agendas in self-management and, in particular, to ignore patients' own strategies for managing a chronic condition and to discount experiential knowledge (15, 16).

Other models of self care support preceded and have continued to develop and be evaluated alongside the self care support training adopted by the EPP (17). To be more effective, support for self care requires two key changes in thinking:

- A whole systems perspective that engages patient, practitioner, and service organization

- Widening the evidence base to acknowledge recent research on the way in which patients and professionals respond to long-term conditions

The Whole Systems Informing Self-Management Engagement (WISE) approach[3] has been developed by our group in Manchester to improve self care support by considering:

- Patient s' self care needs, experience, and knowledge related to the management of their condition

- Engagement and involvement of health professionals

- The fit with services and access arrangements in health care systems

Support for self care clearly has the potential to improve the quality of care for people with LTCs. All levels of the health care system could benefit from change to create the context in which self care can thrive.

Endnotes

1 Further details of the research and references for publications can be obtained from the NPCRDC website: http://www.npcrdc.ac.uk/ProjectDetail.cfm?ID=117.

2 Effect size for self-efficacy = 0.44, and for energy = 0.18. In general an effect size of 0.8 is high, 0.5 is medium and 0.2 is small.

3 http://www.npcrdc.ac.uk/The_WISE©_approach_to_supporting_self_care_in_the_NHS.htm

Coventry University Applied Research Centre Health and Lifestyle Interventions: Learning from Co-Creating Health

Louise M. Wallace

Introduction

Co-Creating Health (CCH) is a unique initiative (described in Chapter 13) with programmes acting via patients, clinicians, and services to create system wide support for self-management. The evaluation was commissioned from a team at the Applied Research Centre Health & Lifestyles Interventions at Coventry University. They have expertise researching health services management, and complex behavioural interventions for supporting change in the organization of services, the practice of clinicians and in self-management by patients.

The evaluation is both summative and formative in nature. Both approaches use a mix of methods including interviews and surveys of patients and health care professionals, observation of the three delivery programmes within the initiative and analysis of health service data.

The summative evaluation focuses on what the programme achieves in relation to improving patient reported and clinical outcomes as well as health service utilisation. Currently, data collection is underway using surveys, interviews, and health service data.

The formative evaluation, which seeks to understand how the programme is being implemented, uses observation and interviews to surface the assumptions and/or underlying 'theory' of CCH. The evaluation team are testing ways to share findings with the demonstration sites to help them reflect on their progress.

At the time of writing, the CCH programme is nearing its mid point. Consequently, the learning that can be shared is primarily from the process evaluation on two components of the programme. A range of methods is being used, but we are able to share insights from interviews with tutors and participants from the co-delivered Self-Management Programme (SMP) and the Advanced Development Programme for clinicians (ADP) that took place in the early half of the programme. This learning has been of benefit to those delivering the programme and it is hoped that it may be of use to others in developing self-management support beyond the traditional methods of lay-led programmes.

Co-production

In a clear departure from most self-management programmes worldwide, and particularly in the UK, the concept of co-production is central to CCH. One example of *co-production* being demonstrated within the programme is through the patient and clinician tutors working together to co-deliver the SMP and ADP course.

While previous evaluations of programmes delivered either by a patient *or* clinician tutors have found little or no difference in participant outcomes (18–20), the co-production model is an novel aspect of CCH. In this chapter, we explore the learning so far about co-delivery by lay and clinician tutors.

One of the challenges for CCH is to train clinicians to engage in co-production in both their clinic consultations, and in co-delivery of programmes with lay tutors. The model of lay-led programmes may challenge clinicians' beliefs about what will be effective. Wilson (21) reported that health care professionals demonstrated a lack of engagement with the Expert Patient Programme (EPP) and a lack of acceptance of the validity of a lay-led self care support programme. Lay-led programmes may also challenge the traditional communication repertoire of clinicians. Newman et al. (22) have argued that health professionals tend to use verbal persuasion and information giving, both of which are poor at building patients' self-efficacy for self-management. One of the recommendations in a King's Fund working paper (23) was that health professionals should attend training programmes to learn how to develop and foster self-management skills among their patients.

The evaluation explores the extent to which the combined style of delivery of courses by tutors helps to achieve a positive motivation by participants for applying the learning they achieve through attending the SMP and ADP courses.

According to Ryan and Deci's (24) 'Self-Determination Theory', learning outcomes depend largely on the social context in which the teaching is delivered. This applies both to teaching designed to change a clinician's practices, and to teaching designed to change a patient's health-related behaviours. Content can be delivered in ways that are 'autonomy supportive' or 'controlling'. Autonomy supportive social contexts facilitate self-determined motivation to learn, while a controlling style promotes learning only due to the external demands, usually with much poorer outcomes. An autonomy supportive style learning climate can be described using 3 dimensions:

- ◆ Autonomy support: the tutor provides participants with choice and meaningful rationales, minimizes demands.
- ◆ Structure: the tutor sets goals, makes expectations clear and provides adequate and well-timed feedback.
- ◆ Interpersonal involvement: the tutor dedicates psychological resources, such as time, energy, and affection to the group.

In the section below, we assess how far the teaching approaches used within Co-Creating Health constitute 'autonomy-supportive' learning climates, and therefore have the potential to deliver the desired learning outcomes.

The Self-Management Programme for patients – learning from the process evaluation

The Self-Management Programme within Co-Creating Health teaches specific self-management techniques, including personal behaviour and emotion focussed coping, as well as using group processes (social support, role modelling by a patient and clinician tutor) to effect cognitive and behavioural changes in participants. Unlike the general EPP, it is designed for groups of patients with the same clinical condition and the programme content has been modified to include condition specific content.

Each of the sessions is co-delivered by a clinician tutor, who works locally in the relevant pathway of care, and a patient tutor who has experience of these services.

It is too early at the time of writing to report the outcomes, however, the design of the programme was based on the hypothesis that this programme would lead to:

- An improvement in patient activation (defined as self-management skills, knowledge and confidence)
- An increase in the use of self-management techniques (e.g. positive and active engagement in life, health directed behaviour, skill and technique acquisition, constructive attitudes and approaches, self-monitoring and insight)
- Reductions in psychological distress (anxiety and depression)

The interviews undertaken following early courses show promising improvements in confidence to self-manage:

'I've had COPD now for almost four years now … it's obviously had an effect on my life … going on the course has certainly made me a bit more confident about dealing with certain aspects of it'.

SMP graduate

Patients reported that they gained knowledge not only from the formal instruction components of the course and from the clinician tutor, but also from the social aspects of exchanging with other patients their shared experience of living with a particular long term condition. Feeling more educated about their long term condition, patients were then more able to accept the condition and to have greater confidence in their ability to cope:

'Well I think it gave me a bit more confidence in what was wrong with me, because if you've got mysteries, you don't know how to cope with mysteries. But going on that course, it gave you more information and I felt generally that that's what's helped me'.

SMP graduate

The evaluation team tested whether tutors delivered in accordance with the Self-Determination Theory. This allowed us to assess how the style of the course may impact on the motivation of participants to learn and apply the learning to their lives.

We rated the patient and clinician tutors' style on three scales:

- Tutor's Autonomy Support
- Tutor's Structure
- Tutor's Involvement

Preliminary findings suggest that there is no significant difference between the scores of clinician tutors and patient tutors on any of the subscales in relation to the SMP. The ratings of the two tutors positively correlate, suggesting that the delivery skills are balanced and both tutors are contributing to motivating self-management in patients.

We interviewed patients who had been on the SMP as well as those who were delivering the course. All were positive about the co-production model of SMP. They recognized the different skills that each of the tutors brought to the SMP, valuing the patient tutors' life experience of living with a LTC, but also appreciating the clinical expertise of the clinician. Themes which came out of the analysis of these early interviews include the suggestion that the co-delivery model encourages continued attendance of the SMP as the clinician tutor's presence increases the value placed on the course by some patients:

> 'Well I just thought the professional person, well she was professional, she knew her job. I don't know, maybe it was just more reassurance than anything else'.
>
> SMP graduate

Some patients reported that having a clinician as co-tutor breaks down boundaries between patients and clinicians. We suggest that this represents added value for patients from the co-production model of delivery.

Although SMP graduates explicitly stated that the clinician and patient tutors were equal, the language used by SMP graduates to describe the tutors differed. Patient tutors were often described as 'the volunteer', whereas the clinician tutor was described as 'the one taking the course', the 'main coordinator', or the 'paid tutor'. This may be at least partially explained by clinicians being paid to deliver these courses (through their contracted salaries), but not paying patients to tutor courses: this was observed and commented upon in conversations between tutors in front of course attendees.

A further point we are exploring, which the CCH programme as a whole is seeking to address, is the ambivalence expressed by some clinician tutors about their role:

> 'I don't know why I was there as a healthcare professional because I didn't do anything that a lay person couldn't have done. You could have had a lay person doing that. Why was I there? I have no idea'.
>
> SMP clinician tutor

This suggests that there is not yet a fully shared understanding of the hypothesis and aims of the co-production model, namely that it has an inherent value in so far as it provides a model to course participants of clinicians and patients working together in equal partnership. To achieve the objectives of CCH, we recommend that further work is needed in our demonstration sites to ensure that this underlying model of learning is shared, understood and enacted by all tutors.

The Advanced Development Programme for clinicians – learning from the process evaluation

The Advanced Development Programme for clinicians (ADP) seeks to train clinicians to apply a range of communication and behaviour change skills in their consultations with patients with long-term conditions. It is co-delivered by a clinician and a lay tutor. Our early results are drawn from interviews with attendees and tutors on the first 2 courses at each site. These findings reflect initial experiences from the very first year of the programme. The mode of delivery of the courses has changed in response to feedback from participants and demonstration sites.

Our interviews with clinician participants from the courses explored how they have applied their skills. We found that most often there is an incremental improvement in behavioural skills they were already using.

> 'Applying the ADP … is just giving patients the opportunity to think more, and being realistic about setting some plans with a patient, a sort of management plan that they can follow as well as other health professionals can look at, rather than trying to make decisions and make everyone better'.

Clinician tutor on both the ADP and SMP

One of the clinician tutors however pointed out the need for further support after the course in order to maintain and refresh these skills:

> 'beyond those skills which are around good communication and agenda setting and dealing with empathy, when it comes to goal setting and goal follow-up, …. I anticipate that without the ongoing support of an individual (tutor).… I think these skills are likely to just become less and less used'.

Clinician Tutor

In response to the recognition of the need for greater post-course follow-up, in year 2 of the initiative almost all of the sites have been offering action learning sets. One of the Co-Creating Health sites has also put in place additional support for clinicians, such as 1–1 coaching designed to help them to maintain the use of the new skills within their practice and to support them with the challenges that arise.

Clinician participant responses to a post ADP survey of the first and second series of courses showed that the style of the clinician tutor was rated as successfully supporting autonomous learning by providing choices and a good structure for learning. However, the clinician tutor's input was somewhat less successful at supporting autonomous learning by providing interpersonal involvement with participants on the part of the tutor (e.g. by providing affection).

In the first two series of courses, it was found that the patient tutors scored significantly lower on all of these dimensions. While this may reflect the style of contribution, it may also reflect the lower levels of tutor activity and perhaps perceived role of patient tutors. We explored this issue by direct observation of the delivery of a sample of sessions. The preliminary non-participant observations of early ADP programmes showed that the patient tutors' role was often confined to participating in role play activities as patients, which was contrary to the initial design of the programme in which – like the Self-Management Programme – clinician tutors and patient tutors took equal co-delivery roles.

We explored the views of clinicians about the impact of the co production delivery of ADP in interviews with participants. Some were supportive of the role of the lay tutor:

> 'It gets the perspective right for a lot of clinicians and [builds their] understanding of patients' emotions when they come for the consultation'.

> Clinician ADP graduate

However, several course attendees and a clinician tutor, who were interviewed, made comments that seem to reinforce that the visible activities of the lay tutor were largely constrained to role playing patients or providing a patient perspective:

> 'I suppose through the other aspects of Co-creating Health I've seen the impact it can have to have patients or lay individuals in a room, and it's generally very positive. But in the end we are here teaching a skill set, and that's what it's about, and I would anticipate that ADP tutors with or without a lay tutor can deliver that'.

> Clinician Tutor

We have shared these findings with the sites and those delivering these programmes. Our observations are not surprising in the light of the fact that many clinicians have not had the experience that their more junior colleagues will now have, of experiencing training by lay people as patients during their pre-qualification training. It may also be a role that some patients are uncomfortable with initially. Since these observations, the patient tutor role has been strengthened with the aim of achieving a greater balance of delivery within the

ADP, including greater patient tutor visibility and leadership. We will evaluate future courses to see if a more co-equal co-production model emerges.

The Service Improvement Programme – learning from the process evaluation

The Service Improvement Programme (SIP) aims to engage clinicians and patients in developing healthcare support systems that embed joint agenda setting, goal setting and goal follow up within routine clinical processes. The quality improvement approach used within the programme includes incremental change and measurement of impact – such as patients' confidence in self-management goals set within consultations. At the time of writing, all sites have begun to experiment with introducing simple aids to improve the use of agenda setting, goal setting, and follow up support tools in consultations. For example, a clinician who attended the ADP is introducing new forms of letters to patients to support their patients' self-management plans. A colleague in the same team commented:

> 'I think very much about structuring a consultation around agenda setting and the shared agenda setting around specific goals. And I think that that's really come out quite obviously in the doctors' letters. So two of the consultants, their letters are brilliant. They already were pretty good but, you know, I was reading one of the consultant's letters, I saw a patient for follow-up from her appointment with him, and it was just brilliant, the letter was brilliant'.

> Clinician graduate

Others have noticed effects on their own practice:

> 'I've produced an agenda sheet that I'm trying out with patients which offers a menu of options of things to talk about.'

> Clinician graduate

However, others are more cautious in judging whether these new systems were embedded fully:

> 'We are using agenda setting, goal setting and goal follow-up in my clinic ... we are trying to use these in our day to day practice but there hasn't been a huge trend of it'.

> Clinician graduate

It is likely that for widespread and sustained implementation that system 'prompts' and feedback systems will need to be incorporated.

Cross-site level – learning from the process evaluation

Learning is encouraged between sites and at the level of the whole programme in many ways, including a shared extranet, monthly teleconference calls with the whole programme team focussing on each site and National Forums. There have been 3 of these so far and a further two are planned. They afford sharing of experience as well as learning from international experts and patient leaders. The first Forum was structured by The Health Foundation, but sought to introduce patients' perspectives and ensure cross site learning:

'This was excellent … putting patients and their stories at the centre'.

Anon. participant

Subsequent Forums have steadily shifted towards more site input on design and delivery and, in early 2009, attempted to involve patients as co-designers more directly. It is apparent from our participant observation that for many patients, clinicians and managers, these events challenge their established notions of their roles, and it has required careful thought and planning to ensure equal participation at all levels.

For others, the Forum had potential extrinsic value. The invitation of influential stakeholders, such as the site Trusts' CEOs, was important to maintaining the profile of CCH locally, as well as access to resources. One person stated the main benefit had been:

'Bringing one of our commissioners to the table so that she grasps more fully the extent to which commissioners need to consider all of what needs to be in place to support self-management. The CEO meeting … where we talked about how we need to … be more explicit re anticipated benefits to patients, clinicians, boards'.

Anon

Conclusions: capturing the learning for self-management programmes

We have explored some of the impacts of the programmes, and tested the value of co-production in delivery of the early courses. The co-production model has perceived benefits, but whether there are distinctly different and necessary contributions from the clinician and patient tutors will require further testing, in particular when the programmes are fully delivered by local site clinicians and patients rather than by national experts. It can be argued that including a clinician tutor helps to position self-management within mainstream health care, so moving beyond what has historically been the realm of the largely unpaid voluntary sector. However, the necessary contribution of clinician tutors and whether they add value beyond that of a dual patient delivery model, has not been established at this stage. The additional costs of salaries, which if extended to patient tutors would further increase cost, will be important variables for any future cost–benefit analysis of the co-production model.

The participants we interviewed expressed many positive benefits from attending the SMP and ADP courses, and those who experienced as clinicians the combination of the Advanced Development Programme and the Service Improvement Programme were able to see how the overall ethos of CCH – to create an integrated approach to building self-management support as part of the fabric of the service may begin to take shape as the initiative matures. There are strands of evidence that the sum of CCH is more than the value of its programmes. The evaluation will contribute to achieving this aim by continuing to capture, analyse, and give feedback on the process of delivery and the outcomes achieved.

References

1. Buszewicz M., Rait G., Griffin M., et al. (2006) Self management of arthritis in primary care: randomised controlled trial. *BMJ* 333(7574): 879.

2. Kennedy A., Reeves D., Bower P., et al. (2007a) The effectiveness and cost effectiveness of a national lay led self care support programme for patients with long-term conditions: a pragmatic randomised controlled trial. *Journal of Epidemiology and Community Health*. 61: 254–61.

3. Griffiths C., Motlib J., Azad A., et al. (2005) Randomised controlled trial of a lay-led self-management programme for Bangladeshi patients with chronic disease. *British Journal of General Practice*. 55: 831–7.

4. Richardson G., Bojke C., Kennedy A., et al. (2008) What outcomes are important to patients with long term conditions? A discrete choice experiment. *Value in Health*. 12(2): 331–9.

5. Kennedy A., Gately C., Rogers A. (2005) Process Evaluation of the EPP – Report II: Examination of the implementation of the Expert Patients Programme within the structures and locality contexts of the NHS in England, National Primary Care Research and Development Centre, University of Manchester.

6. Bandura A. (1977) Self-efficacy: Toward a unifying theory of behavioral change. *Psychological Review*. 84(2): 191–215.

7. Kennedy A., Rogers A., Crossley M. (2007b) Participation, roles and the dynamics of change in a group-delivered self-management course for people living with HIV. *Qualitative Health Research*. 17(6): 744–58.

8. Wilkinson RG. (2001) *Mind the Gap: Hierarchies, Health and Human Evolution*. Yale University Press.

9. Department of Health (2005). New perspectives. *Expert Patients Programme Update*. 14: 15.

10. Reeves D., Kennedy A., Fullwood C. et al. (2008) Predicting who will benefit from an Expert Patients Programme self-management course. *British Journal of General Practice*. 58(548): 198–203.

11. May C. (2006) Editorial: The hard work of being ill. *Chronic Illness*. 2: 161–62.

12. Sanders C., Rogers A., Gately C., Kennedy A. (2008) Planning for end of life care within lay-led chronic illness self-management training: The significance of 'death awareness' and biographical context in participant accounts. *Social Science & Medicine*. 66(4): 982–93.

13. Gately C., Rogers A., Sanders C. (2007) Re-thinking the relationship between long-term condition self-management education and the utilisation of health services. *Social Science & Medicine.* **65**(5): 934–45.

14. Pilgrim D., Rogers A., Bentall, R. (2009) The centrality of personal relationships in the creation and amelioration of mental health problems: the current interdisciplinary case. *Health.* **13**: 235–54.

15. Rogers A., Kennedy A., Nelson E., Robinson A. (2005) Uncovering the limits of patient centredness: a qualitative investigation of implementing a self-management trial for chronic illness. *Qualitative Health Research.* **15**(2): 224–39.

16. Wilson PM. (2001) A policy analysis of the Expert Patient in the United Kingdom: self care as an expression of pastoral power? *Health and Social Care in the Community.* **9**(3): 134–42.

17. Kennedy A., Rogers A., Bower P. (2007c) Support for self care for patients with chronic disease. *BMJ.* **335**(7627): 968–70.

18. Cohen J., Sauter S., DeVellis R., DeVellis B. (1986) Evaluation of arthritis self-management courses led by laypersons and by professionals. *Arthritis and Rheumatism.* **29**(3): 388–93.

19. de Weerdt I., Visser A., Kok G., de Weerdt O., van der Veen E. (1991) Randomized controlled multicentre evaluation of an education programme for insulin-treated diabetic patients: effects on metabolic control, quality of life, and costs of therapy. *Diabetic Medicine.* **8**(4): 338–45.

20. Lorig K., Feigenbaum P., Regan C., Ung E., Chastain RL., Holman HR. (1986) A comparison of lay-taught and professional-taught arthritis self-management courses. *Journal of Rheumatology.* **13**(4): 763–7.

21. Wilson PM. (2008) The UK Expert Patients Programme: Lessons learned and Implications for Cancer Survivors' Self Care Support. *Journal of Cancer Survivorship.* **2**: 45–52.

22. Newman S., Cooke D. (2008) Conclusions. In: Newman S, Steed E, Mulligan K (editors) *Chronic Physical Illness: Self-Management and Behavioural Interventions.* Maidenhead, UK: McGraw-Hill.

23. Corben S., Rosen R. (2005) Self-management for long term conditions: Patients' perspectives on the way ahead. www.kingsfund.org.uk.

24. Ryan RM, Deci EL (2000) Self-determination theory and the facilitation of intrinsic motivation, social development and well being. *American Psychologist.* **55**(1): 68–78.

Chapter 15

'Hard talk': What do we really know about the benefits and value of self-management course provision?

David G. Taylor

There is nothing new about self care and self-management, defined in terms of the actions taken by people – either alone or with others' support – to preserve or restore their own health and overcome disabilities and associated challenges. Throughout history, individuals, with their families or other members of their communities, have had to cope with illness and handicaps as best they can, given their personal values and aspirations and the realities of the social and material worlds surrounding them.

Even as recently as in the 1800s, when the health professions we now know were forming and modern medical technologies were starting to become available, there remained a strong heritage of personal and village or street level collective self-reliance. Our Victorian predecessors had strong appetites for not only self care remedies (which were on occasions of very dubious value) and 'self improvement' manuals but also for supporting local philanthropic works and establishing mutual benefit organizations.

The developments of the twentieth century, and in particular the creation of the NHS and the wider welfare state after 'Hitler's war', to a degree lessened the perceived need for personal expressions of social solidarity. They may also have to an extent – and for a time – have reduced public and professional awareness of the central role that individuals must often play as the primary producers (as distinct from just the co-producers) of their own health. The reality, however, is that even in modern societies people deal with many of their health related problems with little or no formal help. Indeed, developments such as mass access to the internet may be increasing the frequency with which this occurs.

It is understandable that professionals such as doctors, nurses, and pharmacists, anxious to contribute to the wellbeing of others and build further their own careers, may come to feel that health care is something they 'do' to patients, rather than with and for active individuals who are in control of their own lives. There is evidence that traditionally oriented professionals can underestimate, and sometimes ignore altogether, the importance of 'lay' coping strategies and skills. Taken too far, even well meant paternalism threatens the self-respect and self-reliance that for many – if not all – people in many – if not all – societies is a core component of well-being and the experience of 'healthiness'.

Likewise political leaders – especially in the UK, where the creation and running of the NHS has arguably played an unusually significant role in maintaining their legitimacy – may also have come to see health and health care as 'services' they provide to populations, as distinct from benefits that individuals and communities in large part generate for themselves. Yet with the increasing prevalence of long-term conditions and the emergence of supporting people with them as a dominant task facing all developed country health and social care systems (coupled with factors such as globalization, and the economic challenges now affecting mature economies with costly welfare systems) there has since the start of the 1980s been a partial rediscovery of the importance of self care.

It is against this background that this chapter offers a discussion based largely on the important insights provided by other contributors to this book. It explores the extent to which the increasing emphasis on self care and self-management in the UK health policy can be seen as a substantive advance, as distinct from something that is of value to a limited number of enthusiastic individuals but unlikely to have a major impact on the overall population. It also considers whether or not developments such as the introduction of the Expert Patient Programme have been in part driven by a desire for cost cutting or even a concealed wish to undermine the standing of professionals such as GPs, as opposed to a positive desire to improve health outcomes and foster desirable changes in professional practice and social attitudes.

Effective, well-informed, self-management can play an important role in improving the outcomes of virtually every form of preventive and ameliorative health care. Yet against this, exaggerated claims for self-management/self care programmes could prove to be a barrier to the general acceptance of useful practice and patient support improvements amongst not only health professionals but also those using health services.

Witnessed value

The evidence assembled in this book addresses self-management at a number of levels. Christine Cupid, Barbara Hogg, and Carol McNaughton, for instance, describe attending courses such as Challenging Arthritis and the EPP, and their personal journeys from relative social isolation and feelings of defeat in life through to a recovered position and ongoing involvement in the support of others facing problems similar to those they successfully solved.

Other writers, from Jean Thompson to Jane Cooper, Mike Osborn, Patrick Hill, and Julie Barlow, describe aspects of self-management course development, delivery, and evaluation; while Ayesha Dost and David Colin Thomé provide additional insights into policy formation and implementation processes. Similarly, Natalie Grazin's contribution likewise provides a useful reminder of the integrated approach to chronic care developed by Ed Wagner in Seattle, which is reflected not only in the Health Care Foundation's work but also the NPCRDC's Whole System Informing Self-Management Engagement (WISE) model.

These and other contributors in many instances describe experiences which have helped to determine the value they place on self-management support. They include not only overcoming losses of confidence caused by distressing forms of ill health, and becoming better able to cope with problems such as continuing pain or limited mobility, but also taking part in management and research activities which have proved to be highly significant in individuals' subsequent careers and identities. The development of self-management courses and other forms of health service user support and representation have, for example, been important in the personal stories of Kate Lorig and Roy Jones, as well as – at an impersonal, functional, level – for the populations in which their individual contributions have helped to generate welfare gains.

Personal witness and belief has an inherent integrity which is often intimately associated with the factors driving the behaviour of people involved in health and social care provision and use. It provides the *pathos* needed to translate *logos* and *ethos* into a valued world, and so deserves to be heard carefully in any system genuinely seeking insight into the highest priority needs and concerns of those it serves. Sensitivity to subjective realities is central to sustainable political decision making and policy making.

The importance that Bob Sang and Jean Thompson attach to 'lay leadership' in the context of self-management support, and more broadly to the balancing of institutionalized professional power and authority with independent service user representation and advocacy, is a theme relevant to this point. Such concerns are given additional strength by the warnings from contributors like Julie Barlow and Roy Jones, which draw attention to the fact that well meant attempts to measure the tangible benefits that individuals gain from attending self-management courses can fail to take into account social changes ultimately resulting from their provision. Yet in the final analysis, these last as they affect areas such as the relationships between health service users and professionals, may prove far more important than the immediate individual benefits of self care support, albeit that the complexity of community development processes often makes determining causality inherently uncertain.

How effective is self-management support and how durable are its benefits?

At the same time, it is also obviously important to avoid confusing phenomena such as faith, hope, and individual commitment with dispassionate, quantitatively-based, analyses of what does or does not work in a cost-effective manner to achieve the defined goals in given settings. At worst, a failure to be rigorous in this context could risk distorting the measurement of public interests by viewing policy options through the screen of personal hopes, ambitions, and fears.

Standing back from the transformational gains that some who have been on programmes such as, say, Lorig's CDSMP and British EPP courses have clearly enjoyed, the research findings reported by authors such as Julie Barlow, Anne Kennedy, Anne Rogers, and Kate Lorig indicate that relatively modest (albeit by NICE standards cost effective) gains in variables such as 'energy levels' and 'self efficacy' more typically result from attending general self-management courses. Clinically provided rehabilitative and training courses in areas such as HIV, asthma, CVD, and diabetes self care appear to more effective in enabling individuals to acquire specific competencies in areas like medicine taking, even if these might not in the long-term be as productive as helping individuals to enjoy raised health related self-efficacy (and/or become less depressed) and so go on gaining new skills indefinitely.

There is good evidence that for many of the people – most often women – who choose to join and subsequently attend short self-management courses, these are likely of genuine yet limited value. As David Colin-Thomé's analysis indicates, NHS investments of public resources in their provision are justifiable. But they do not offer 'miracle cures', and there are a number of caveats that should be added to this finding. One, as Anne Kennedy makes clear, is that intermediate outcome measures such as increases in measured self-efficacy should not uncritically be taken to 'prove' that end point health outcome improvements are being achieved.

Likewise, even though 'mastery' and allied experiences can promote self-efficacy gains (defined as increased context specific self confidence that may enable individuals to learn and adapt more rapidly than would otherwise be the case) this does not inevitably mean that those who have been on self-management courses enjoy benefits that endure over long periods of time, as compared with what would otherwise have been the case. It is possible that self-management interventions in many instances serve to accelerate the development of coping mechanisms and self care skill acquisition, rather than opening the door to changes which would otherwise have been permanently impossible.

Implications for professional practice

In her interview with Roy Jones, Kate Lorig argues that although the fact that the NHS has developed an approach-based on her work which has helped to give it world-wide credibility, it was possibly unfortunate to have adopted the term 'the Expert Patient Programme'. Lorig says this helped to fuel the perception that supporting self-management somehow involves excluding or denigrating the contributions of health professionals. In some instances, political interventions apparently aimed at limiting the power of the medical profession to challenge central decision makers could have strengthened this impression. Kate Lorig is also critical of the cost of the bureacratized British system of self-management course assessment.

Other commentators disagree, either because they do not think that the language of the EPP has discouraged professional involvement or because they regard challenging traditional professionalism as desirable. Strands of debate as to whether or not it was right for the NHS to seemingly 'take over' support for self-management from organizations such as Arthritis Care run, both overtly and covertly, throughout much of this book. So too do questions about whether or not professionals (and modern scientific medicine) are part of the problem we are seeking to overcome, as opposed to a key to the self-management solution waiting to be unlocked.

It is possible that for some people and groups the personal and group conflicts at the heart of such issues will never be fully resolved. Nevertheless, thinking like that underpinning the NPCRDC's WISE approach and the Health Foundation's Co-creating Health initiative implies that promoting self-management and care need not, and should not, be seen as a threat to professionalism. It may rather be regarded as part of a process of evolutionary adjustment that will help health care systems as a whole cope with growing workloads in more efficient and appropriate ways, and allow patients and professionals to build more productive relationships.

If this last view is accepted then understanding the significance of the interventions such as those now offered in the UK by the EPP Community Interest Company and other 'third sector' bodies, represents an important opportunity for all health professionals and educators. Regardless of the potential of self-management (along with relevant skills training, and if required self care support services embodying limited elements of long term community nursing and/or social care) to reduce the costs of health care or effect the progression of conditions like arthritis, gaining insight into why self-management principles and goals are so highly valued by committed people ought to be of considerable value to anyone seeking to live well with long-term illness.

Will investing more in self-management cut health care use?

Research from the US suggests that enabling people with long-term conditions to attend self-management courses can lead to reduced use of health services and cost savings. Similar claims have on occasions been made is this country. It is argued that 70–80% or so of individuals with long-term conditions can, with relatively limited support, 'self care'. If true, this might enable more costly resources to be concentrated on complex and high-risk cases.

However, there is as yet no substantive research demonstrating that the provision of self-management courses has led to health service cost reductions in this country. One possible reason for this is that the British approach to primary and community ('ambulant') care provision already allows for greater efficiency and flexibility than is often the case in the US, where the proportion of GDP spent on health services is twice the UK figure.

Given this, some commentators may be tempted to question aspects of the policies described by Ayesha Dost and David Colin-Thomé. But the evidence presented in this book indicates that service quality and outcomes can be cost effectively enhanced via the provision of self care support, in return for relatively small increases in expenditure. The point to stress is, improving cost effectiveness is not necessarily the same thing as reducing overall costs.

In the English health care environment, the genesis of direct public involvement in self-management via the EPP dates back to 2000, and the start of a period of unprecedented NHS expenditure increases. Between that year and 2009, an additional 2% of GDP has been channelled into health services and salaries. This is comparable to the entire GDP share growth enjoyed by the NHS in the half century between 1950 and 2000. Seen from this perspective it is relatively unlikely that simplistic, short or even medium term cost saving goals underpinned the political instigation of the EPP. A genuine desire for quality improvement, coupled perhaps with a parallel desire to communicate to critics of increased public spending on health that new investment has not been made wastefully, is a more plausible interpretation.

Conclusions – self-management and social change

As societies grow richer and more educated, the people living in them typically enjoy increased life expectancies and better protection from infection. But this imposes costs related to the long-term damage caused by increased access to the 'fruits of plenty', such as tobacco, alcohol, motorized transport, and fatty foods. Alongside ageing, this has driven rising absolute levels of chronic illness.

As populations become wealthier, they also come to expect higher standards of (universal) service provision and treatment safety, alongside more choice and increased personal autonomy. The late twentieth century 'rediscovery' of self-management in countries like the UK can be seen as an integral aspect of this complex process of 'care transition', which is in one way or another reflected in every chapter of this book. The social changes associated with the twenty-first century modernization are promoting further developments such as a growing requirement for new types of service relationship between health care providers and users.

Initiatives such as the establishment of the EPP–CIC can be partly seen as a response to changing demand. Yet, at the same time, access to self-management programmes of all types is likely itself to have a modest but nevertheless a material impact on public and patient expectations and perceived responsibilities. The conclusion offered here is that their emergence is both a result and an engine of changing patterns of health aspiration and care demand.

The capacity of individually oriented self care support to promote phenomena such as an increased level of population 'engagement' in health improvement, or alter patients' experiences of limiting, painful and otherwise distressing long-term conditions, should not be over-stated. But within the wider context of ongoing care transition, science-based pharmaceutical and other forms of therapeutic advance and rising community expectations that people, despite potentially disabling disorders, should be able to achieve fulfilment in and positive control over their lives, it has a significant part to play in improving health care and health outcomes.

An important challenge to overcome in the next decade is to help both service commissioners and care providers understand fully this reality. Taken together, the contributions in this book show that self-management support offers a way of promoting further health gains consistent with the interests of the Treasury and health professionals, as well as those of patients, families, and community groups seeking as best they can to achieve their goals and overcome the challenges of illness and mortality. Kate Lorig observes that God helps individuals and communities who help themselves. She is almost certainly right, albeit that those who help others will also always have a vital role to play.

Key References

Porter R. (1997) *The Greatest Benefit to Mankind. A Medical History of Humanity from Antiquity to the Present.* London: Harper Collins.

Taylor D., Bury M. (2007) Chronic illness, expert patients and care transition. *Sociology of Health and Illness.* **29**(1): 27–45.

Department of Health (2001) *The Expert Patient: A New Approach to Chronic Disease Management for the 21st Century.* London: Department of Health.

National Primary Care Research and Development Centre (2008) *The Wise Approach.* Manchester: NPCRDC.

Chapter 16

Which way is forward?

F. Roy Jones

Ever since the success of the initial arthritis course, the Stanford self-management courses have had to bear a weight of hope and expectations. While the Arthritis Foundations of the English-speaking world were gaining experience with delivery, researchers were busy exploring the theories that might adequately account for the phenomena observed. On the other hand, health service planners, profoundly concerned about a possibly exponential growth in demand, wondered if these courses might be a way to transfer at least some of the burden of illness back to the patient. In short, this work has always had policy implications and these have been constantly explored.

In the preceding chapters, the many ways in which NHS thinking and assumptions pervade the UK's national subconscious has become increasingly apparent. A further illustration might help. In the early days of Challenging Arthritis, a Scottish nurse tutor lost her job due to OA hip because it prevented her from doing the necessary lifting tasks. She did not view this problem as a 'disability' to which legislation might apply, but as a 'disease', and she therefore left her job on medical grounds. A self-management course equipped her to reconstruct her life. Becoming a tutor she wrote, 'I had to un-learn so much of my nursing training. I had been taught to look at patients as needy. Now, I had to see people as resourceful'. In acute medicine, the patient's resourcefulness is mostly irrelevant. In long-term conditions it is both essential and, quite fundamentally, different. Here, the patient's need to be treated as a whole being predominates and attempts to deliver services as if the condition were acute, seem all too often, doomed to fail. A diabetes nurse specialist told me, 'I am always making contracts with my patients but they always break them'. She was profoundly frustrated and disappointed that it was so rare to meet a patient wanting to make the life-style changes necessary to assert control over his/her life with diabetes. Indeed, she added, many who urgently needed to make life-style changes for their health and longevity would agree to anything to get their medications.

Several versions of the pyramid devised since 1999 by Ayesha Dost when at the DH have become familiar. They make the point that the vast majority of health care is self care and health professional input is necessarily infrequent. The implication is that the quality of self care is of major importance, and we know from her Chapter 10 that self-management courses contribute to that capacity. The more severe the condition(s), the more involved the individual becomes with professional health services (Fig. 16.1).

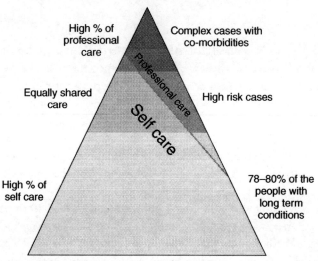

Fig. 16.1 Self care among people with long term conditions. (Original: 1999)

Source: "Our health, our care, our say" Department of Health White Paper, January 2006

As the author, I claim no expertise about Kaiser Permanente (KP), the US integrated managed care organization, now working in 9 states. (Incidentally it also holds the largest number of Stanford licences.) There is a striking omission in the UK papers reporting its work. KP's 2004 paper, Evolution of Health Education[1] has some special importance. No commentator doubts KP's financial sophistication, so I was impressed to observe that this paper reports that every aspect of its health education programme has been accompanied by a detailed Return on Investment (ROI) analysis. Unsurprisingly, the calculation details are not readily available; however, it can be assumed that the costings offset clinician and treatment costs against educational inputs. Fig. 16.2 is an attempt to summarize the import of the chart 'Educational Stratification Levels'. Further, when new organizations sign up for KP services an assessment is made of the health literacy of the community from which their workers and families are drawn. In areas of low-health literacy, KP volunteers conduct courses to raise the level so that they can make optimal use of their services. While accepting that this is a very American model, it justifies serious examination especially as it asserts the need for health competencies in the general community and that education is a root contribution.

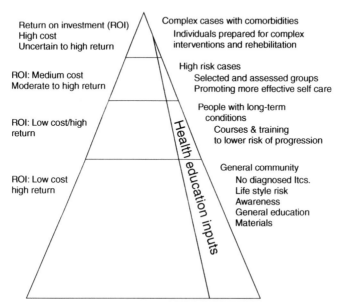

Fig. 16.2 Kaiser Permanente Health Education Stratification.

It is apparent that both in the US and the UK the desirability and potential national health benefits (including societal cost reductions) have yet to be recognized. Each KP centre offers, where it is offering services, a very substantial range of education programmes and it is clear that the style of these varies with the educational need of the patients involved. This raises a profound question, 'Is the UK similarly failing to deliver a national strategy, offering in its place a plethora of supported but limited services?' It is not as though there is no consensus about what informed commentators want for our citizenry. We want everyone to make choices that are good for their immediate and long-term health on the basis of evidence and their own skill and good sense. However, clinical and demographic evidence suggests this is far from universally the case, leaving the methodological question to be answered. I am suggesting that understanding ourselves and our health deserves greater attention by educationalists deploying modern methods. Modern approaches include harnessing the power of peer learning, and the use of training methodologies when these are the most effective. The experiences of developers, especially Kathy Hawley and Andy Turner, demonstrate this. In short, NHS services to people with long-term conditions want and need a community of empowered patients. The absence of work on lay competencies from the agenda of Skills for Health seems to me to unfortunate.

Natalie Grazin refers to Ed Wagner's work (see her references) that has informed Stanford thinking for many years. UK pharmacy practice has examined the language and practice of compliance and concordance. There may well be a spectrum of response here. In acute conditions and events, compliance is necessary. However for a long-term concordant pattern, it is the engagement, a partnership with clinicians that is required. Living with a long-term condition means experiencing the processes Patrick Hill and Jenny Newbould have described. Indeed, living with increased risk is part of living with long-term conditions. This has to be addressed and then subordinated to ongoing life purposes. That is concordance and consequently congruent with self-management approaches.

The interpersonal dimension serves to illustrate the complexity of the educational task to be addressed. The individual's learning style is hugely influential. Most people learn quickly from people facing similar issues, perceived as being like themselves. This is one of the great strengths of the lay-led ideal. Its power to release energy is a potent resource and it would be folly to waste it. The need to overcome any alienation this has engendered needs to be addressed (see Barbara Hogg, Chapter 3 and Jean Thompson Chapter 5). Whoever we are, we share common experiences when we face common diagnoses. For health professionals, the experience is, for many, no less laicising. In the North West, there have been courses recruited exclusively from among health professionals working in a PCT.

David Taylor has fully explored the ongoing debate about evidence and the policy context, in Chapter 15. We share a concern for the academic security of the programmes and his contextualizing the many contributions in this book is masterly. I have two major nagging concerns.

Two nagging concerns

The first is that some influential self-management practitioners and developers have been content to continue delivering courses knowing that their senior managements conceived what was being done differently. Too often I have heard, 'So long as they'll let us do what we want (deliver self-management courses) it doesn't matter that management doesn't fully understand it'. This has sometimes amounted to collusion with the fundamental misunderstanding that these courses are about imparting a body of knowledge and, in the longer term, confusion between commissioners and providers. In reality, self-management courses are more like working for your sailing or gliding qualifications. Yes, there is stuff you need to know, but you also have to show that you can use that information when you go solo on the lake or make that first circuit of your local airfield. The course is about becoming self-reliant, knowing the resources that are available and being confident that you can organize your life to retain the maximum possible control over challenging chronic disease. Now, from management's viewpoint, this outcome seems very much what they hoped for; articulate people coping better with their conditions. But it is not the same. Perhaps, Bob Sang has captured it by saying self-management is not about meeting need, but about reawakening people's ambition: life opening up in a new way, not shutting down. This also seems consistent with Mike Bury's thinking as outlined by Jenny Newbould in Chapter 3 and described elegantly by Patrick Hill in Chapter 7. But it should be added, this was not the purpose of many paternalist services: they were about sympathy and kindness. Self management is about that reawakening.

The concept of a population capable of 'implementing personal choice' is readily understood by people living and working in environments where new information regularly influences the day's work choices. For most it is more complex: here is a more basic example. Supporting self care is often said to be supporting people's good habits such as twice daily teeth brushing. If you ask a dentist how many of their patients do this, the answer seems encouraging. Ask how many know how to brush their teeth and maintain good oral hygiene, and the answers are depressing. Another example: In the Australian pre-study for their national pilot, the thought was explored of using long-term care plans in general practice with GPs providing diagnoses, and nurses providing the regular contact. At the feedback conference, community-based clinicians pointed to a conceptual error. The assumption had been made that demand for health professional support correlated with disease severity. They reported that this was not the case. The better correlation was with the self-management skills of individuals. Some people with substantial difficulties nevertheless cope brilliantly, while some, with clinically minor issues, are almost helpless. That was when their Department of Health and Ageing went looking for a generic course and found Stanford's.

The second nagging thought is allied to the first. Why don't we see in the research results the transformations that motivate the volunteer course tutors to continue delivering this work? It is seeing people grow and transform that keeps these people going, not course completions or the possibility of remuneration (see Julie Barlow's Chapter 14 p 138 on Lay Tutors). Naturally, self-management courses are not for everyone, there are people in all walks of life who naturally use their heads to first understand what's going on, select the best course of action, and then, crucially, move to action. Such people attending a course may not get much out of it directly beyond discovering they are not alone and can be a resource to others. Kate Lorig discusses this in her foreword and suggests that numbers and the averaging process reduce the apparent affect. Could it also be that because managements, not having understood the process, commission research that cannot identify such results, looking for behavioural change and health gain when the scope is wider? Another illustration: The very first time the arthritis course was discussed at one of Arthritis Care's regional councils an older woman, a course graduate, stood up and said something to this effect, 'I've had arthritis for 25 years but I went on the course. It's not for me. I hadn't much to learn about arthritis. I think it would be better for younger people'. Her course tutors were speechless. Since the course she had re-joined her church choir and was getting up in the mornings and relating to her family. This was a changed person to the resigned woman with painful hips who came to the course reluctantly and now, belatedly, relates well to her doctor. To research such changes, very different protocols are needed. The standard off the peg research instruments that give credibility to research reporting may not be appropriate. My nagging thought focuses down to, why has there been no *educational* research? We do know that learning new life skills can transform lives.

Natalie Grazin and the Health Foundation are surely correct when they point out that, in England, systemic change in the public perception of health without the NHS is an awesome task and it is more than attitudinal: it has structural dimensions. Ayesha Dost has pointed out how little time people spend with health professionals and consequently how great a proportion of care for people with long-term conditions is self care (see Fig. 16.1). It is within this larger umbrella that self-management courses find their place. However, in the emerging community of agencies that deliver self-management courses to an agreed standard, both in local communities and within the NHS, there is a ferment of innovation. The authenticity of such work is illustrated in Elizabeth Bayliss's contribution (see Chapter 6). That said, I have to emphasise, that in my experience of third-sector conversations, the scale, depth, and complexity of this apparently simple realization is wildly underestimated. The thinking associated with acute conditions is deeply institutionalized. To move away from this requires that the patient pathway for people with long-term conditions be visibly different. Such diagnoses carry the need for motivated effort on the part of the patient not just compliance. This is not about patients becoming 'medical' beyond a basic competency level, it is about the self-management objectives, rehearsed once again below, much of which is best explored in community-based groups where peer learning potential abounds. An oblique illustration: recently, in a trials committee, we spent much time discussing patient consent and compliance, fall off rates, and the support needed by patients to persist with the intervention being studied. There was very little about why a patient might choose this new regime. It is an optional treatment, what's to discuss? Patient motivation was simply not relevant. Now, I know these researchers to be kind and thoughtful human beings, so their contacts will be handled with humour and warmth. That is not my point. My point is that teaching adults without reference to their hopes and ambitions misses something crucial that is likely to influence outcomes (not least that they learn most efficiently from each other). Projects can fail to achieve most needed characteristic: developing the resourcefulness of patients.

Below the public horizon, many initiatives are in progress. Stanford is being asked to license new community agencies. The Quality Institute is resourcing PCTs, the voluntary sector and new social enterprises are developing their own programmes. It is apparent that the final shape and place of self-management in the UK firmament is not yet clear.

Conclusions

1. On learning a diagnosis of chronic disease, a different framework needs to be entered where the contribution of the patient is prepared and supported with professionally designed educational programmes, and by general practice with a facilitative rather than a prescriptive style. This implies engaging the central reality, namely, there are a great many people with long-term conditions, not now successful self-managers, who need to be equipped to use their own heads to:

   ◆ Solve problems

   ◆ Make decisions

   ◆ Use available resources

   ◆ Form partnerships with health care providers (and others)

   ◆ Move to action promptly

   Establishing a strong sense of control is a determinant of good outcomes.

2. The capacity of individuals to manage their own learning varies hugely. Good teachers, facilitators, and trainers all equip their students to do this. An ambition from the early days is now, (gratifyingly), reappearing in the Health Foundation material: every encounter with a health professional should build an individual's competence to care for themselves. So far, Skills for Health has not been briefed to focus on the aching void of health competencies in the general community.

3. Making self-management available might well provide a tool that can equip communities to use their health and social care providers appropriately, not in compliance, but in the co-creation of healthy communities. The sales point is that they equip people to benefit from community resources,

including other courses, and use information sources effectively. As social care and health care are brought closer together in policy and delivery systems, the need for common approaches grows. It may not cut service utilization, but it might well enhance its effectiveness.

4. The EPP–CIC is structuring itself to operate in a marketplace of course providers. For all its power and urgent drive to become the predominant national provider, I remain to be convinced that this is self-management training as we've defined it. I do not doubt that some staffs are delivering self-management courses authentically, but I discern an unresolved tension between these people and management.

There is no question that there is a growth in demand for medical care from people of all ages with long-term conditions. There is a special question about the preparedness of the older community to take on the self care tasks in later years. As Bette Davis said, 'Getting old ain't for cissies'. Self-management can surely develop many forms. To be authentic I want to hold to the criteria at the head of this section. It changes people's vocabulary of concern from sympathy to supporting activity.

The End is Not Yet

Richard Gutch warned many years ago that institutionalizing self-management might distort its purposes. In the UK, I think we have witnessed that happening as people have corseted it to fit their fashionable agendas. I remain no less committed to its value and am delighted by the variety of forms in which it is now appearing. This is not about blind adherence to the excellent work shared round the world by Kate Lorig and her colleagues: it builds on it. It is about the capacity of communities to relate to the sheer numbers of people in their midst living with long-term conditions and doing well. That simply cannot happen without community activists and their essential partners, the health professionals.

I would like to think reading this book has made the task a little easier to comprehend and engage. It's not rocket science. Great insight does not have to be complex.

Endnotes

1 Health Promotion Practice (2004) DOI: 10.1177/1524839903258730, *Health Promotion Practice* 5: 20.

Martha A.V., Nancy K., Ronald B.N., Frayne R., Mei Ling Schwartz

The Evolution of Health Education: The Kaiser Permanente Southern California Experience.

The free online version of this article can be found at www.sagepublications.com.

Index